ROYAL COMMISSION ON
THE NATIONAL HEALTH SERVICE

Patients' Attitudes to the Hospital Service

Research Paper Number 5

LONDON: HER MAJESTY'S STATIONERY OFFICE

ISBN 0   11   730115   9

Foreword by the Chairman

The Royal Commission on the National Health Service was appointed in May 1976 with the following terms of reference:

"To consider in the interests both of the patients and of those who work in the National Health Service the best use and management of the financial and manpower resources of the National Health Service."

The terms of reference cover the NHS in England, Scotland and Wales as well as the parallel services in Northern Ireland.

This is the fifth in the series of Research Papers we have published dealing with important aspects of our remit. As with previous Papers our object is to stimulate and inform public discussion of the issues with which it deals.

The views expressed are those of the author and not of the Royal Commission.

A. W. Merrison
December 1978

Patients' Attitudes to the Hospital Service

A survey carried out for the Royal Commission on the
National Health Service to find out about the experiences
and attitudes of users of the hospital service.

Janet Gregory

Social Survey Division
Office of Population Censuses and Surveys

ACKNOWLEDGEMENTS

Although only one name appears on the cover of this report, a study such as this is the result of the work of many people. In particular I should like to thank Elizabeth Breeze, Dympna Waldron, Stella Chidley and David Lloyd of our technical branches, Lesley Sanders of research branch, Jeremy Harbison of the Survey Unit, Northern Ireland Office, and Christine Farrell, research officer with the Royal Commission for their help and advice in the design and the analysis of this study.

I am also indebted to all the interviewers who worked on the study and to all the patients who so willingly gave up their time to talk to us.

NOTES TO TABLES

(i)   — indicates no case fell into this category.

(ii)   * denotes less than 0.5%.

(iii)   [] denotes number given, not percentage: base figure usually too small.

(iv)   small variations between tables in the base figures for the same sub-group are due to varying numbers of 'no answers' having been excluded.

(v)   for the sake of simplicity and consistency tables have been headed 'Men' and 'Women' even when they include children under 14. It should be remembered however that for child patients information was collected from parents, and where opinions were sought, it is the views of these parents that are recorded in the tables.

Contents

1.0 Introduction

1.1 Background to the survey

In December 1976 the Commission asked the Social Survey Division of the Office of Population Censuses and Surveys to explore the possibility of carrying out a national survey of patients' attitudes to and experiences of National Health Service hospital services.

A study commissioned by the four Health Departments in the UK, examining the accessibility to patients of the primary health care services (provided by doctors, dentists, pharmacists, opticians, district nurses, health visitors and chiropodists) was already in hand.[1] However since this particular study was concerned solely with primary health care provision it would not provide any information on the experiences and opinions of people using the hospital service. Moreover the study was too far advanced for additional questions to be incorporated to meet this need. Therefore the possibility of conducting an enquiry specifically designed to cover hospital experience was discussed.

The survey of patients' attitudes to the hospital service was formally commissioned in April 1977. A small pilot and feasibility study was carried out in July 1977 and the interviews for the main stage survey were conducted between November 1977 and January 1978. The full report was presented to the Royal Commission in August 1978.

1.2 The survey design

The sample[2]

The overall aim of the survey was to find out about people's experiences of, and attitudes towards the hospital service provided by the National Health Service; the views of patients using the outpatient service as well as those who had been admitted as inpatients were to be covered by the survey.

Initially there seemed to be a number of possible ways in which the two samples, one of outpatients and one of inpatients, could be selected. The most obvious source was to use the records held by the hospitals themselves; this had the particular advantage that people would be able to talk about a recent hospital experience. However the use of hospital records was rejected principally because there was insufficient time to inform both the hospital authorities, at regional, local and individual hospital level, and individual consultants, of our proposals and to obtain their agreement to the sampling and interviewing taking place.

Taking a random sample from the general population was also decided against. From published statistics it was known that only about one in ten of the general population had been to hospital as an outpatient or casualty in a three

---

1. Access to Primary Health Care: Jane Ritchie and Ann Jacoby: HMSO awaiting publication.
2. Full details of the sample design are given in Appendix I.

month period, and only about one in seven had any inpatient experience in a 12 month period. It would therefore have been both expensive and time consuming to have asked interviewers to have first identified people with recent outpatient or inpatient experience from a list of addresses before going on to a full interview. A postal enquiry to identify outpatients and inpatients prior to a personal interview was also rejected since it would take too long to administer and process.

Social Survey Division does however conduct a multi-purpose on-going survey, the General Household Survey (GHS), in which a sample of about 14,500 addresses are contacted over a 12 month period, and everyone aged 16 and over in the household interviewed. Started in 1971 the GHS includes core questions on aspects of housing, education, employment and health, and the 1976 and 1977 questionnaires included a question which asked whether anyone living at the sampled address had attended *"as a patient the casualty or outpatient department of a hospital (apart from ante- or post-natal clinics)"* in the three complete calendar months prior to the date on which they were being interviewed.

The GHS also asks one member of the household, usually the head of the household, or housewife, whether, if at any time a Government department required further information on any of the topics covered in the GHS interview, they would be willing for us to recall and interview any member of the household again. Thus we had a potential source of people with *outpatient* experience.

However a sample of people with inpatient experience was not as readily available. The 1976 GHS questionnaire had included a question asking about inpatient experience in a three month period, but in 1977 the question referred only to people with chronic conditions. Since the number of inpatients identified in 1976 was too small for our purposes (because of the three month reference period) and the 1977 questionnaire would produce a very special sample of inpatients, it was therefore decided to add a special 'trailer' question to the second and third quarters of the 1977 questionnaire to identify anyone in the household with recent inpatient experience, whom we could then call back upon and interview. [3] [4]

A three month reference period for inpatient experience would not yield adequate numbers over only two quarters of GHS, so it was decided to extend the reference period to include any inpatient experience in the 12 month period prior to interview. This was expected to yield, over the two quarters, about 1,000 inpatients, which after allowing for non-response to our own survey would be a minimum number suitable for the analyses envisaged; it was also about the

---

3. Details of the workings of the GHS trailer system are available on application from the GHS Unit, Social Survey Division, OPCS, 10 Kingsway, London WC2B 6JP.

4. It was already too late to include a trailer question to be asked of the sample approached in the first three months of 1977, and we could not extend coverage into the final quarter of the year if we were going to be able to call back on these people in January 1978; the processing of the GHS information and the production of address lists for this survey would not be ready in time.

maximum number that we felt we would be able to interview and process in the time available.

As regards the size of the outpatients sample, the limiting factors were our own resources and the time available. It was decided to include anyone interviewed on GHS during the whole of 1976 who had outpatient experience: an estimated 2,500 informants. This would be an adequate number for analysis and about the maximum number we could hope to deal with in the time available.

The question used on the 1976 GHS schedule to identify 'outpatients', and the 1977 'trailer' question designed to identify people with inpatient experience are reproduced in Appendix II.

Northern Ireland sample

The Commission particularly asked, for the sake of complete coverage, that Northern Ireland be included in the survey. It was pointed out in initial discussions that the limited sample size meant that it would not be possible to make any regional comparisons, or to compare Northern Ireland with the rest of the United Kingdom.

The GHS is not conducted in Northern Ireland and therefore special arrangements had to be made to obtain the samples of inpatients and outpatients: a small postal enquiry was carried out as a preliminary stage to interviewing. A short questionnaire and covering letter were sent in August 1977 to a sample of 341 addresses selected from the Northern Ireland Valuation lists. This number represents the correct proportion of addresses that would be included in one year if the GHS were conducted in Northern Ireland. People were asked to record the name, sex and age of everyone who lived at the address and to indicate on the postal form anyone who had been to hospital as an outpatient or casualty at anytime since 1st May 1977, and also anyone who had been in hospital overnight or longer since 1st August 1976. Reminder letters were sent to non responders at two and again at four weeks after the initial mailing.[5] The documents used, together with copies of the reminder letter are reproduced in Appendix II.

The response to the postal was extremely good; replies were received from 281 (82%) of the original 341 addresses. On the postal form 76 people indicated that they had been to hospital as an outpatient or casualty since 1st August 1977, 55 people indicated that they had been in hospital as an inpatient overnight or longer since 1st August 1976, and 28 people recorded both outpatient and inpatient experience in the specified periods.

It is important to note that at this stage the samples from Northern Ireland were not comparable to those selected for interview in England, Wales and Scotland. In order to achieve comparability and therefore to allow the results

---

5. The administration of the postal enquiry and the subsequent interviews with patients in Northern Ireland were carried out by the staff of the Social Survey Unit of the Statistics and Economics Unit at Stormont. We are extremely grateful for their help and co-operation.

from Great Britain and Northern Ireland to be added together to produce data for the United Kingdom, a number of corrections needed to be applied to the Northern Ireland sample.

Firstly, the reference period for outpatient experience needed to be defined as a three month period, and that for inpatient experience as a 12 month period. This was done at the interview stage; anyone contacted whose only experience was outside the specified periods was ineligible for a full interview.

Secondly, it was necessary to take a subsample of one in two from the inpatient sample in Northern Ireland. It will be remembered that the initial selection of 341 addresses in Northern Ireland was proportional to the total number of addresses selected in *one year* for the GHS in Great Britain. However, because the inpatient sample in Great Britain was selected from addresses contacted over a *six month* period, the Northern Ireland sample needed to be subsampled for comparability; this was done at the analysis stage.

Finally, 28 people indicated on the postal form that they had been both outpatients and inpatients since the dates given. (It will be remembered that the two samples in Great Britain were independent, being selected from data obtained in different years by the GHS). In Northern Ireland such people should have been interviewed in respect of both experiences, with the inpatient interviews then being subsampled as outlined above; it was decided however to interview solely in respect of the inpatient experience. Since the number of such people is very small, this decision is unlikely to have affected the nature of the outpatient data overall.

The interview questionnaires

Two questionnaires were developed for use on this study; one for patients who had attended hospital for treatment as outpatients or casualties and one for patients who had attended as inpatients. Each questionnaire dealt principally with the five main areas in which the Commission had expressed a particular interest:

    i.   the provision of hospital transport for patients to and from the hospital;

    ii.   the length of time spent waiting for a first outpatient appointment or as inpatients for a hospital bed;

    iii.   the provision of facilities and amenities in the outpatient clinics for patients and those accompanying them, and similarly the facilities in the hospital wards and rooms for inpatients;

    iv.   communication between hospital doctor and patient;

 and v.   the degree of privacy afforded to patients.

In addition, the questionnaires included short sections concerned with the special provisions in hospitals for young children, with patients' attitudes to the hospital staff they met, and, for inpatients only, questions about the arrangements the hospital had for visiting, and about arrangements for care and advice after the patient was discharged.

Apart from collecting factual information about the hospital service that patients had experienced, it was particularly important that in addition to knowing how satisfied patients were with the existing provisions, the Commission should know how concerned patients were if some aspect of the service was seemingly inadequate, or some amenity lacking. Without this information there would be no indication of the relative importance to the patient of any improvements that might be considered.

It was decided *not* to ask patients about their satisfaction with their actual treatment and with the standard of medical care they had received, for two reasons: firstly there was no objective standard against which to set their answers and secondly, it was felt that the patient's own views on his treatment would not be a sound basis on which to make recommendations for changes or improvements.

The interview sample and response

WHO WAS INTERVIEWED:
Personal interviews were carried out with men and women aged 14 and over who had been identified as having attended hospital as an outpatient or casualty (apart from visits to ante or post-natal clinics) in a specified three month period, or who had been inpatients overnight or longer at any time during a specified 12 month period. Where the patient was a child aged under 14, a proxy interview was taken, usually with the child's mother. Proxy interviews were not accepted in other instances, for example when the 'patient' was currently too ill or had died since the original GHS interview (or postal enquiry), since a large proportion of the questionnaire asks for the patient's own opinion of the hospital service that he or she had experienced.

Neither the GHS nor the postal enquiry in Northern Ireland identified people attending hospital as private patients; as our brief was to find out the views of patients on the hospital service provided by the National Health Service, the questionnaires relating to the 22 inpatients and 20 outpatients who were found at the interview stage to have attended hospital as private patients, have been withdrawn and excluded from the analysis and discussion that follows in this report.[6]

THE RESPONSE
Interviewing took place between 1st November 1977 and 31st January 1978. In both Great Britain and Northern Ireland the response to the survey was good, especially when it is remembered that in Great Britain these people had already been interviewed previously as part of the GHS, and that the selection of names and addresses which were now part of our outpatient sample had originally been made from the 1976 Electoral Register. Table 1.1 below shows a summary analysis to response at the interview stages in Great Britain and Northern Ireland.[7]

---

6. Patients who were referred to the hospital by a private doctor or consultant, but who subsequently received NHS hospital treatment have *not* been excluded.

7. Further details of response are given in Appendix I.

Table 1.1 Response rates and non-response at the interview stage for the two samples in Great Britain and Northern Ireland separately.

	Inpatient sample				Outpatient sample			
	GB		NI		GB		NI	
Set sample	911		83		2674		76	
Ineligible for interview	36		20		118		31	
	No	%	No	%	No	%	No	%
Total eligible sample	874	100	63	100	2556	100	45	100
Total non response:	83	9	4	6	294	12	1	2
refusals	38	4	0	0	101	4	1	2
non contacts	45	5	4	6	193	8	0	0
Total interviews	791	91	59	94	2262	88	44	98
Withdrawn	1		0		19		0	
Private patients	22		0		20		0	
Total for analysis	797 (after subsampling NI sample)				2267			

'Ineligible for interview' included cases where the patient had died, and where the date of the outpatient visit or inpatient spell was found to be outside the specified reference periods. The proportions of ineligible patients in the Northern Ireland samples are much greater than for the Great Britain samples since the specific reference periods were not given on the postal form but only disclosed at the interview stage.

'Refusal' included patients who were too ill or too confused to be interviewed although they had been contacted, as well as patients who did not agree to take part in the survey.

The interviews withdrawn included further cases identified as ineligible at the coding stage where the outpatient visit or inpatient spell was outside the reference period, and cases where the patient had not visited a hospital but had attended, for example, a Local Authority Day Centre, or Family Planning Clinic.

1.3 Plan of the Report

Throughout this report the results from the interviews with the two sample groups, outpatients and inpatients, are discussed separately, under common chapter headings and after general introductory remarks, and it should be remembered that although in some cases the two sample groups were asked identical questions, they are two independent samples and therefore the results from the two samples cannot be added together. The chapter that follows describes the main characteristics of the two samples and then the report goes on to deal with the areas of principal interest to the Commission: chapter 3 is concerned with waiting times—for appointments and hospital admission. Chapter 4 describes the methods of transport used by patients to get to and from the hospital and in particular their use of, and satisfaction with, transport provided by the hospital. Chapters 5 and 6 look at the facilities and amenities provided at the hospital in outpatient departments and for inpatients in the wards and other parts of the hospital. We then go on in chapter 7 to look at the way in which the hospital appointment system was working. In chapter 8 we look at various aspects of privacy and chapters 9 and 10 discuss communications and relationships between patients, doctors and other hospital staff. Chapter 11 describes the arrangements made for discharging inpatients from hospital and the help that was given, or was needed, once they were home, chapter 12 deals with parents' attitudes to their child's stay in hospital and chapter 13 is a note on dissatisfaction with the NHS hospital service in general.

2.0 The characteristics of the sample

This chapter describes the characteristics of the two samples of patients who were interviewed. The age, sex, marital status and working status composition of the samples are shown together with an analysis showing how many patients had other people in their household dependent on them and hence particularly likely to be affected by their going into hospital or attending hospital as an outpatient. These are the main factors which may help explain many of the differences in experiences and attitudes that were found, and which are described later in this report. These factors have therefore been used as the main variables in the analyses.

Having described the personal characteristics of each sample we then look at the patient's experience of the hospital service, as an inpatient or as an outpatient as appropriate, in the relevant reference periods, and also at any previous or more recent experience which may have affected their responses to our questions.

2.1 The inpatient sample

Interviews were achieved with 243 men and 457 women aged 14 and over who had been in hospital as inpatients overnight or longer in a 12 month period.[8] In addition one of the parents, usually the mother, of 64 boys and 33 girls aged under 14 who had also been inpatients in this period was interviewed. Table 2.1 below shows the numbers and proportions of men and women 'inpatients' in various age groups.[9]

Table 2.1 **Proportions of men and women inpatients in various age groups.**

Age groups	Men		Women		All inpatients
	Nos	%	Nos	%	%
0—4	26	8	12	3	5
5—9	27	9	15	3	5
10—13	11	4	6	1	2
14—16	11	4	1	*	2
17—24	25	8	73	15	12
25—34	24	8	128	26	19
35—44	32	10	54	11	11
45—54	49	16	61	13	14
55—59	18	6	36	7	7
60—64	31	10	18	4	6
65—74	39	13	50	10	11
75 and over	14	4	36	7	6
Base: all inpatients=100%	307		490		797

8. In Great Britain the reference period was any 12 month period between 1 April 1976 and 30 September 1977, in Northern Ireland the period was from 1 August 1976 to 1 August 1977.

9. The term *inpatients* will be used in this report to refer to informants living in private households who had been in hospital overnight or longer in the 12 month reference period. It does not refer to informants' status at the time of interview.

If this data is presented in another way—table 2.2 below, it can clearly be seen that there are considerable variations both between the overall proportion of men and women and between the proportion of men and women in the various age groups; for example, of the 797 men and women interviewed one in four was a woman aged between 17 and 34, while less than one in ten of those interviewed was a man in the same age group.

Table 2.2   Proportions of those interviewed in different age groups: men and women inpatients.

Sex	Age groups						
	0—9	10—16	17—34	35—54	55—64	65 & over	All ages
Men %:	7	3	6	10	6	7	39
Women %:	3	1	25	14	7	11	61
All inpatients %:	10	4	31	25	13	17	Base=100%=797

Four main differences are apparent from the table; the greater number of women compared to men, the predominance of women aged 17-34, as previously mentioned, the excess of male children over female children particularly under the age of 10, and the greater proportion of elderly ·women compared with elderly men. These differences were expected; the greater number of women overall and in particular the greater number of young women is largely accounted for by maternity cases, (93 women were interviewed whose sole experience of being in hospital in the 12 month period was to have a baby) and the greater proportion of elderly women reflects the differences in the age structure for men and women in the general population. However the differences we found in our sample between the proportion of boys aged 0—9 and the proportion of girls aged 0—9, although well established and documented by other sources, is not fully understood.[10] Table 2.3 below shows the marital status of the men and women interviewed, and as would be expected from what has been said previously, married women account for the largest group—over 40% of those interviewed.

Table 2.3   Proportions of those interviewed who were married, were single, or were widowed or divorced: inpatients

Sex	Marital status			
	Married	Single	Widowed/divorced	All
Men %	22	14	2	39
Women %	43	9	9	61
All inpatients %	65	23	11	Base=100%=797

The next chapter considers how convenient the date of admission was for the patient and any inconvenience waiting for a hospital bed caused, and it may be of interest to compare the views of patients who were in employment with those who

---

10. See for example Report of the Hospital Inpatient Enquiry DHSS and OPCS, HMSO Report on the National Child Development Study, and Cartwright A, Human Relations and Hospital Care Routledge & Kegan Paul.

had no job. The table below shows the composition of the sample in terms of working status.

Table 2.4 Working status of men and women inpatients

Working status	Men		Women		Men and women
	Nos	%	Nos	%	%
working: full time	129	42	66	14	25
part time	4	1	72	15	10
unemployed	8	3	5	1	2
retired/off sick	90	29	118	24	26
housewife	—	—	180	39	23
in education—aged 16 and over	2	1	0	—	*
under 16	74	24	34	7	14
Base: all inpatients=100%	307		475		782

Again when looking at admission procedures and waiting times, and later in the report when patient satisfaction with, for example, visiting and after care arrangements is discussed it might be useful to consider the extent to which the patient had other members of their household dependent (not only financially) on them. It is not possible to define precisely all conditions of dependence from household composition information, nor, without a great deal of questioning and analysis, discover what help might be available to the dependants of inpatients. We know for example that some neighbours will take over responsibility in caring for children, and relatives or neighbours may take children into their own homes, or come to live in the family home while the patient is away. We therefore defined just four relationships between patient and dependants, which were the ones thought most likely to be affected by the patient going into hospital: these and their frequency distribution in the sample are set out below.

A: The patient is a non working mother with one or more children aged under 11 in the household: 148 cases
We decided that only children under 11 would be regarded as dependent on their mother (the patient) and only then if the mother did not have a job.

B: A two-person household where the dependant was aged 75 or over: 16 cases
Probably either a two-person pensioner household, or a household where a younger person, the patient, was living with someone considerably older, for example daughter and mother.

C: The patient is a child (under 14) whose mother is not working and who has brothers or sisters aged under 11: 46 cases
In such situations the concern may be over who can look after the other children while the mother is visiting the child in hospital.

D: The patient is a child (under 14) whose mother is working: 34 cases
Caring for the child after he has been discharged from hospital may present problems to a working mother, but it should be noted that only 15 of these mothers had a full time job, the rest were working only part-time.

10

Hospital inpatient experience

The General Household Survey had originally collected brief information about each spell that the patient had been in hospital during the 12 month reference period.

These details were checked by the interviewers working on this survey and as can be seen from the table below 85% of patients had only had one inpatient spell in the 12 month period.

Table 2.5 Number of inpatient spells and number of conditions treated during the 12 month reference period

No. of conditions treated	No. of inpatient spells in 12 month period				All inpatients	
	1	2	3	4 or more	Nos	%
1	678	66	11	5	760	96
2	—	29	2	—	31	4
3	—	—	3	—	3	*
4	—	—	—	1	1	*
All inpatients	678 (85%)	95 (12%)	16 (2%)	6 (1%)	Base = 795 = 100%	

It can also be seen from the table above that over two thirds (70%) of the patients who had been in hospital on more than one occasion during the 12 month period had received treatment for the same condition on each occasion, so that overall, 96% of the patients interviewed had received inpatient treatment for only one condition over the 12 month period.[11]

Further analysis showed that very similar proportions of men and women (86% and 84% respectively) had had only one inpatient spell, but that as table 2.6 below shows there was some indication of differences between the various age groups.

Table 2.6 Proportions of men and women in different age groups who had been into hospital on more than one occasion in a 12 month period

No. of spells in hospital	Age groups					
	0–16	17–34	35–54	55–64	65 & over	All ages
	%	%	%	%	%	%
1 spell	92	85	87	80	86	85
2 spells	7	12	11	15	12	12
3 or more spells	1	3	2	5	2	3
Base: all inpatients=100%	109	250	194	192	50	795

11. It should be noted that we have relied on the patient's own assessment as to whether or not all their inpatient spells related to the same condition.

Amongst the youngest age group (0 to 16) less than one in ten had been into hospital on more than one occasion during the 12 month period but this proportion rose to one in five amongst patients aged 55 to 64.

The *'interview spell'*

Generally in the interview we wanted to confine ourselves to asking the patient about their experiences and reaction to one particular spell in hospital: the *interview spell*. Where there had only been the one inpatient spell in the 12 month reference period, then this was the occasion that was asked about; in the 15% of cases where there had been more than one inpatient spell in the 12 months, we asked only about that spell which had occurred earliest in the reference period. While in the interview we deliberately asked the patient to comment on one particular spell in hospital, we nevertheless realise that it is likely that the experience of earlier or subsequent stays may have coloured their opinion, especially where the treatment had taken place in the same hospital and for the same condition. Table 2.7 below shows the proportion of inpatients who had been into the same hospital for treatment for the same condition on an earlier occasion, and those for whom the inpatient spell under consideration was their first admission to that hospital for that complaint.

Table 2.7 **Proportion of inpatients who had previously been in same hospital for treatment for same condition**

Previous admissions	No. of inpatient spells in 12 month period		
	One	More than one	All inpatients
	%	%	%
first admission	85	73	83
had been in previously	15	27	17
Base: all inpatients =100%	678	119	797

Overall only about one in six inpatients had been admitted on an earlier occasion for treatment for the same condition, although patients who had been in hospital on more than one occasion in the 12 month period were more likely to have had a previous admission for the same complaint than those who had only the one inpatient spell in the 12 months.

By our definition all 119 patients who had been in hospital more than once in the reference period had been in hospital subsequent to the *interview spell*—but less than one in ten (8%) of those with only the one spell in hospital during the 12 month period had been into hospital again for any reason up to the time of interview.

Looking therefore at hospital experience both before and after the *interview spell*—table 2.8 below—it can be seen that two thirds of the patients interviewed had neither been in hospital previously for the same condition, nor had they been back into hospital again since for any reason whatsoever, and hence their opinions of their stay in hospital are unlikely to have been seriously affected by any prior or subsequent experiences. However while it should always be remembered that the views expressed by some patients about a particular spell in hospital are likely to have been coloured by their other inpatient spells, from here on in the report all the experiences and attitudes of inpatients are those related to the one *interview spell* unless specifically stated otherwise.

Table 2.8 Patients' hospital experience prior and subsequent to *interview spell*

Subsequent to *interview spell*	Prior to *interview spell*		
	had been in hospital for same condition	had not been in for same condition	All inpatients
had been into hospital again %	5	16	21
had not been into hospital again %	12	67	79
All inpatients %	17	83	Base=100%=797

Duration of stay in hospital

Over half the patients spoken to had been in hospital on the particular occasion that we were concerned with for seven nights or less, and three quarters had been discharged by the end of the second week. Overall there was almost no difference between the length of time that men had stayed in hospital compared with women. However, as can be seen from table 2.9 below older patients, as one might expect, were more likely to have had a longer inpatient spell than younger patients; well over half of those aged between 0—16 had been discharged by the sixth day, compared with only about a quarter of those aged 55 to 64, and one in five of patients aged 65 and over. Over a quarter of this, the oldest group of patients, were still in hospital at the end of three weeks.

Table 2.9 Duration of stay in hospital for men and women in different age groups—cumulative percentages

Duration of stay in hospital	Age groups					Sex		
	0–16	17–34	35–54	55–64	65 & over	Men	Women	Men & Women
	cum %	cum %	cum %	cum %	cum %	cum %	cum %	cum %
overnight	14	5	3	2	5	7	4	5
2 nights	28	19	12	10	10	15	16	15
3–5 nights	59	51	33	27	20	38	40	39
6–7 nights	76	67	46	36	27	53	52	52
8–14 nights	86	91	75	63	53	75	77	76
15–21 nights	94	97	84	75	70	84	88	86
over 3 weeks— 6 weeks	100	99	94	95	89	94	97	96
over 6 weeks— 3 months		100	99	96	98	98	99	99
over 3 months			100	100	100	100	100	100
Base: all inpatients=100%	109	249	194	102	137	307	487	794

2.2 The outpatient sample

Interviews were achieved with 923 men and 915 women aged 14 and over who *'had attended as a patient the outpatient or casualty department of a hospital'* at any time in a three month reference period.[12] [13] As has previously been pointed out women whose sole experience was as a patient attending routine ante or post natal clinics at a hospital were not interviewed. The parents, again usually the mother, of the 429 children aged under 14 who had also been to hospital as outpatients in the three month period were also interviewed. Three children under 14 were themselves interviewed; the adults who had gone with them to hospital—a school teacher and neighbours, were not available to help us.

Table 2.10 below shows the numbers and proportions of men and women outpatients in various age groups.

Table 2.10   **Proportions of men and women outpatients in various age groups**

Age groups	Men		Women		All outpatients
	Nos	%	Nos	%	%
0—4	60	5	52	5	5
5—9	101	9	83	8	8
10—13	74	6	59	5	6
14—16	61	5	35	3	4
17—24	137	12	92	8	10
25—34	144	12	132	12	12
35—44	138	12	137	12	12
45—54	119	10	137	12	11
55—59	89	8	83	8	8
60—64	65	6	77	7	6
65—74	118	10	142	13	12
75 and over	52	5	80	7	6
Base: all outpatients =100%	1158		1109		2267

On looking at the proportions of those interviewed in different age groups (table 2.11 below) differences were again found but not nearly so marked as for the inpatient group.

Table 2.11   **Proportions of those interviewed in different age groups: men and women outpatients**

Sex		Age groups						
		0—9	10—16	17—34	35—54	55—64	65 and over	All ages
Men	%	7	6	12	11	7	8	51
Women	%	6	4	10	12	7	10	49
All outpatients	%	13	10	22	23	14	18	Base=100%=2267

---

12. In Great Britain the reference period was any 3 month period between 1 October 1975 and 30 November 1976, in Northern Ireland the period was from 1 May 1977 to 31 July 1977.

13. The term *outpatients* will be used in this report to refer to informants who had been to the casualty or outpatient department of a hospital as a patient in the 3 month reference period. It does not refer to informant's status at the time of interview.

14

As can be seen from the table, up to the age of 16 boys were somewhat more heavily represented than girls, but then between the ages of 17 and 64 the proportions of men and women in the sample became very similar, as are the proportions of men and women overall, with finally a somewhat greater proportion of elderly women than elderly men. As with the inpatient sample, these differences are in keeping with the findings of other studies,[14] and although the greater proportion of elderly women compared with elderly men is largely accounted for by the structure of the general population, the literature does not satisfactorily account for the greater proportion of young boys using outpatient facilities compared with girls. Other studies also generally show that between the ages of 17 and 44 more women are attending hospitals as outpatients than men; this is largely accounted for by attendances at ante and post natal clinics which were excluded from this study.

Table 2.12 below shows the marital status of men and women interviewed; unlike the inpatient sample, the proportions of married men and married women in the outpatient sample are similar; there would have been many more married women of course had ante and post natal hospital visits been included.

Table 2.12 Proportions of those interviewed who were married, were single, were widowed or divorced: outpatients

Sex		Marital status			
		Married	Single	Widowed/divorced	All
Men	%	28	20	3	51
Women	%	26	15	8	49
All outpatients	%	54	35	11	Base=100%=2267

Being admitted to hospital can be inconvenient and worrying, other arrangements may have to be made at home to look after dependants, and not all employers are sympathetic to absences from work. Similarly repeated visits to hospital as an outpatient can upset people's domestic and work arrangements adding to their probably already existing anxiety. Appointment times, transport arrangements and the actual length of time spent at the hospital are particular areas likely to be of special concern to patients who have jobs to get back to, or dependants to look after. Table 2.13 below shows the working status of the men and women outpatients, and below the table is given the frequency distribution in the sample of the four categories where the relationship between patient and dependants was thought most likely to be affected by hospital visits (see page 10) for a fuller description of these *categories of dependence*. The age, sex and working status of the patient are the main variables that have been used in the analysis of the data obtained from the outpatient sample, with more rarely, marital status, the categories of dependence defined above and the social class of the patient.

14. See for example, Forsyth G and Logan R: Gateway or dividing line?—a study of hospital outpatients in the 1960s OUP.

Table 2.13 Working status of men and women outpatients

Working status	Men		Women		Men and Women
	Nos	%	Nos	%	%
working: full time	585	51	213	19	35
part time	14	1	151	14	7
unemployed	33	3	12	1	2
retired or off sick	225	19	296	27	23
housewife	—	—	192	17	9
in education					
aged 16 and over	20	2	19	2	2
aged under 16	277	24	218	20	22
Base: all outpatients=100%	1154		1101		2255

Table 2.14 Frequency distribution in the outpatient sample of four groups where the relationship between patient and dependants is most likely to be affected by hospital attendance

Categories of dependence	Nos in sample
A: The patient is a non-working mother with one or more children under 11 in the household	105 cases
B: A two person household where the dependant is aged 75 or over	51 cases
C: The patient is a child whose mother is not working and who has brothers or sisters aged under 11	188 cases
D: The patient is a child whose mother is working	
—full time	55 cases
—part time	128 cases

Hospital outpatient experience

We now go on to look at the patients hospital experience as an outpatient or casualty. The General Household Survey had originally recorded the total number of visits the patient had made to hospital as an outpatient or casualty in a three month period. This information was checked at the beginning of the interview and as can be seen from the table below the majority (60%) of patients had in fact only made one visit to hospital in the three month period; a further 20% had made two visits and 10% three visits. The remaining 10% of patients had averaged at least one visit every three weeks over the three month period. Further analysis (see table 2.15 below) also showed that, having excluded ante and post natal visits from the survey, women were no more likely than men to have made more than one visit to hospital during the period, and that there was only a slight indication that older people made more frequent visits than younger patients.

On looking at the broad reasons for the visits to hospital made by men and by women of different ages, and in particular at the proportions attending as casualty or accident cases, some considerable differences were found. Table 2.16 looks at the earliest visit made by patients during the three month reference period and shows which department was visited on that occasion. For this analysis the departments have been divided into just three groups, the major distinction being between visits to casualty or accident departments, where the patient attended without an appointment (although they may have been given a letter by their GP to take along with them), and visits made as a consultative outpatient, where the patient attended usually following referral by their GP but almost always by appointment. The third category comprised patients who were attending ancillary departments or special clinics such as physiotherapy, X-ray, or psychiatry, for specialist treatment or advice; these patients were again generally being seen by appointment, and following referral from a consultant in some other department in the hospital, or from their GP.[15]

Table 2.15 Number of visits made to hospital in a three month period as an outpatient or casualty by men and women in different age groups

No. of visits	Men and women aged						Men	Women	All out patients
	0—9	10—16	17—34	35—54	55—64	65 and over			
	%	%	%	%	%	%	%	%	%
1	63	67	57	58	62	59	59	61	60
2	21	14	21	21	16	17	20	18	20
3	8	11	11	10	9	10	10	9	10
4—6	4	6	7	6	6	9	6	7	6
7—12	2	1	2	2	4	3	3	2	2
13 or more	2	*	2	3	3	2	2	3	2
Base: all out-patients =100%	295	229	504	529	311	391	1155	1104	2259

15. Most patients were able to distinguish visits to casualty from other outpatient visits but many patients who went to hospital by appointment could go no further than to say they had gone to 'the outpatients' and give brief details of their examination and/or treatment. Without access to hospital or other medical records we must necessarily rely on this sometimes inadequate information.

Table 2.16 Proportions of men and women in different age groups who attended as casualty patients, or consultative outpatients on the earliest visit they made to hospital in the three month period

Patient attended:	Men aged:							Women aged:						
	0–9	10–16	17–34	35–54	55–64	65 & over	All ages	0–9	10–16	17–34	35–54	55–64	65 & over	All ages
	%	%	%	%	%	%	%	%	%	%	%	%	%	%
casualty[1]	42	52	62	35	16	13	39	39	46	33	19	16	17	25
consultative outpatients	54	44	33	52	71	72	52	59	51	59	73	71	69	66
ancillary depts	4	4	5	13	13	15	9	2	3	8	8	13	14	9
Base: all out patients=100%	161	135	281	255	225	99	1156	135	94	224	274	236	146	1109

1. includes 16 men and 10 women who attended casualty but were then admitted to the hospital as inpatients

It can be seen from table 2.16 that men were generally more likely to have attended casualty than women, and that not surprisingly younger patients, and particularly children, are much more likely to have been to casualty departments than older patients.

Of course, as with inpatients where more than one visit had been made to hospital in the three month period not all the visits were necessarily for treatment for the same condition, although only in a very small proportion of cases was the patient attending for treatment for more than one condition; 96% of the patients spoken to had visited hospital in connection with only one condition during the three month period.

Table 2.17 Number of visits made to hospital as an outpatient or casualty, and number of conditions treated during the three month reference period

No. of conditions treated	No. of visits to hospital in 3 month period						All outpatients	
	1	2	3	4–6	7–12	13 or more	Nos	%
1	1356	381	205	123	45	52	2162	96
2	—	50	16	22	8	3	99	4
3	—	—	1	1	1	—	3	*
All out-patients	1356 (60%)	431 (19%)	222 (10%)	146 (7%)	54 (2%)	55 (2%)	Base=2264	=100%

Table 2.17 above also shows that of the 908 patients who had cause to go to hospital more than once in the three months, comparatively few (102—11%) were being treated for different conditions on different occasions; the vast majority (89%) were attending hospital in connection with the same condition on each occasion.

Whereas with the sample of inpatients it had been comparatively easy to ask about the experiences and attitudes of the patient to just one spell in hospital, it was felt that it would be unrealistic to expect people who had been to hospital as outpatients on several, or perhaps many, occasions to be able to isolate and talk about just one particular visit. It was therefore decided to ask patients to talk in general about all their visits to hospital as an outpatient for one particular condition, and as has already been seen 96% of the patients spoken to had in fact, on their various visits to hospital during the three month period, received treatment for only one condition. Where more than one condition was being treated, one was selected at random. The condition to which the patient's visits refer and which are reported on here is called the 'sampled condition', and the table below shows the number of visits made by patients for this condition during the three month period. Since the proportion of patients who had only made the one visit in the entire three months was high, naturally, the proportion who had made just the one visit for the sampled condition was likewise high.

However in the same way as it was felt that the experiences and attitudes of inpatients might be coloured by any inpatient spells they had had either before

Table 2.18 Total number of visits made to hospital as an outpatient or casualty for the *sampled condition* during the three month reference period

Total no. of visits made	%
1	63
2	18
3	9
4–6	6
7–12	2
13 or more	2
Base: all outpatients=100%	2264

or after the spell that occurred during the reference period, so with outpatients, any other visits they had made for the sampled condition prior to, or after the visits we already knew about, might not only colour their views, but also be indistinguishable from the visits made during a three month period. This was in some cases up to 18 months prior to the date of interview. It was therefore decided to ask the patient, when talking generally about his or her outpatient visits for the sampled condition, to include all the visits they had made before, during and after the three month reference period. Where specific information relating to their first visit for that condition was asked for, then that visit could have occurred prior to the three month period, and likewise specific information concerning the last visit, might relate to a visit made the day previous to an interviewer calling.

The table below shows that in 60% of cases the earliest visit that the patient had made to hospital as an outpatient or casualty for the sampled condition in the three month period was in fact the first time they had been to hospital in connection with that condition.

Table 2.19 Proportion of outpatients who had previously attended hospital as an outpatient for treatment for the *sampled condition*

Prior to 3 month period patient had . . .	No. of visits made in 3 month period for sampled condition		
	One	More than one	All outpatients
	%	%	%
not been to hospital	59	62	60
had been to hospital	41	38	40
Base: all outpatients=100%	1417	843	2260

There were however 433 patients who had made only one visit in the three months, and 296 patients who had made more than one visit for the sampled condition, whose earliest visit had been without an appointment; these people were assumed not to be consultative outpatients, but probably casualty or accident cases for whom this visit without an appointment would have been the first they had made for the sampled condition. If these 729 patients are excluded from the analysis then for 41% outpatients who attended hospital with an appointment, the earliest visit made in the three month period was in fact their first visit for the sampled condition.

Overall just over half (53%) the patients spoken to had not been back to the same hospital in connection with the sampled condition since the end of the three month period; this included just ten patients who said they had not yet been back, but they did have a future appointment fixed. Of the 1082 patients who had been again since the end of the three month period 596 (26% of the total sample) were still attending the same hospital at the time of the interview, while the remaining 22% had been back, but had now finished their treatment as far as they could tell.

Looking then at the experience of the outpatient sample overall, summary table 2.20, it can be seen that 27% had only ever made one visit to hospital for the sampled condition, and for a further 15% all the visits they had made in connection with the sampled condition had occurred within the three month reference period. The majority of patients (58%) had made other visits either before and/or after the specified three months, including 26% who were still attending hospital at the time of the interview.

Table 2.20   Patients' hospital experience prior to and after the three month reference period

After three month reference period patient made . . .	No of visits made for sampled condition in the three month period				All outpatients
	one		more than one		
	Prior to 3 month period patient had . . .				
	not been to hospital	been to hospital	not been to hospital	been to hospital	
no further visits %	27	8	15	3	53
further visits %	10	18	8	11	47
All outpatients %	37	26	23	14	Base=100%= 2259

2.3   Summary

Information has been collected from nearly 800 men and women of all ages who were in hospital in Great Britain as inpatients overnight or longer at any time during a 12 month reference period, and from nearly 2,300 men and women who attended as patients the casualty or outpatient department of a hospital (apart from routine ante or post natal visits) at any time in a three month period.

About one in seven of the inpatients spoken to had been into hospital on more than one occasion during the 12 month period, but of these, over two thirds had been receiving treatment for the same condition on each occasion; only about one in twenty of all inpatients had received treatment for more than one condition in the 12 month period. Where a patient had had more than one spell in hospital the patient's experiences and attitudes to the spell that had occurred earliest in the 12 month period were asked about.

One in four outpatients had attended hospital on more than one occasion during the three month period, but overall only one in twenty of all the outpatients spoken to had been attending hospital for more than one condition during that time. Where a patient had been receiving treatment for more than one condition, one was selected at random, and in common with all outpatients, their attitudes and experiences generally to all the outpatient visits they had made for that condition, not just to the visits that had occurred within the three month period, were asked about. In fact, for four out of every ten outpatients spoken to, all their visits for treatment for the sampled condition had occurred during that period, but one in four was still attending hospital for treatment for that condition at the time of interview.

3.0 Waiting times for admission to hospital, or for a first outpatient appointment

One of the criticisms of the National Health Service that is frequently voiced and which is of particular concern is the time that non-emergency patients have to wait either for a hospital bed to become available, or for their first outpatient appointment.

To undertake a detailed study of the time that patients wait to be admitted to hospital from a list, or for a first outpatient appointment,compared for different medical specialties and according to the source of referral was beyond the scope of this study and would probably demand the sort of detailed information on time periods that could be better obtained from hospital records: patients themselves may not be able to give sufficiently accurate information. It was, however, felt to be important to find out whether waiting for a first outpatient appointment or for admission had caused the patient any anxiety or inconvenience, or whether they had been in pain while waiting for a hospital bed or for treatment. In finding out about this, and in looking at whether the patient had waited longer than they had been led to expect, patients were asked how long it had been from when they were first told they would have to attend hospital, or go in for treatment, until they were actually seen or admitted. These 'waiting periods' should therefore be treated with caution and it should also be remembered that they include the period, albeit probably short, between the patient being told admission or outpatient attendance is necessary and their being placed on a 'list'.

3.1 Waiting for admission to hospital as an inpatient

Waiting time for admission may well be different for those who were being admitted for the first time for their particular condition, and for those being readmitted. An attempt was made to standardise the information by asking those who had been readmitted for the same condition to give us details about their first admission for that condition. The numbers involved are given in table 3.1.

Of the 797 inpatients interviewed 661 (83%) had no previous admissions for treatment for the same condition; 97 of these were maternity patients and a further 278 were emergency admissions and these 375 patients have therefore been excluded from the discussion that follows.

Of the 136 patients for whom this was not their first admission, 85 had first been admitted for treatment for the same condition at some time before 1975; we felt that this was possibly too long ago for them to remember accurately what had happened and so they have also been excluded.

Yet a further 25 patients were then excluded as their first admission to hospital had been as an emergency case, leaving 312 patients who had had a bed booked or who were admitted from a waiting list for their first admission. These 312 patients are referred to as 'waiting list patients'.

Table 3.1   Patients who had a bed booked on their first admission

	Nos	%
No previous admissions		
first admission was:		
as emergency	278	35
as maternity case	97	12
waiting list/booked case	286	36
Previous admission		
first admission was pre 1975	85	11
first admission was 1975 or later but as emergency or maternity case	25	3
first admission was 1975 or later as waiting list or booked case patient	26	3
Base: all inpatients interviewed	797	100%

As would be expected generally it was either the patient's own family doctor, or the outpatient department at the hospital they were attending that had arranged the patient's admission. However just under 10% reported that NHS inpatient treatment had been arranged for them by a private consultant or specialist.

Table 3.2   Who arranged for the patient to be admitted to hospital on the first occasion

Admission was arranged by	%	
Patient's GP, family doctor	39	
Outpatient department		
at same hospital where admitted	35	50
at different hospital to where admitted	15	
Private consultant or specialist	9	
Other	2	
Base: all who had a bed booked for first admission=100%	302[1]	

1. excludes 10 patients who could not remember who arranged their first admission

Over a quarter of the waiting list patients were admitted within two weeks of being told they would have to go into hospital, and two thirds of those waiting for a bed had been admitted within three months; 6% did however have to wait 12 months or more for a bed on their first admission. The time taken to admit a patient to hospital is obviously governed by a number of factors, including the urgency with which treatment is required and the number of other patients already waiting for the same treatment—factors which we could not take into account. We did however look at the length of time patients had waited from first being told they would have to go into hospital until they were actually admitted, according to who had arranged the admission. As can be seen from table 3.3 below patients who were already attending hospital for treatment as outpatients were generally admitted quicker than those whose admission was arranged by their GP.

Table 3.3 Length of time from first being told to being admitted for patients whose admission was arranged by their GP, or through the outpatients department of a hospital

Length of time:	Admission arranged by:			All[1]
	GP	Outpatient dept. at hospital	Private consultant	
	cum %	cum %	cum f.	cum %
less than a week	8	15	[7]	15
1 week—less than 2 weeks	17	28	[10]	26
2 weeks—less than 1 month	34	48	[17]	45
1 month—less than 3 months	61	69	[18]	66
3 months—less than 6 months	85	88	[21]	86
6 months—less than 12 months	92	95	[25]	94
12 months or longer	100	100	[26]	100
Base: all who had a bed booked for first admission=100%	117	149	26	298

1. includes the small number of patients whose admission was arranged by some other agency.

Nearly half the patients whose admission was arranged by doctors at the hospital where they were already attending as outpatients were admitted in less than a month, while only about one third of those whose admission was arranged by their GP had been admitted by that time. (We found no differences between those admitted to the same hospital as they were attending as outpatients, and those admitted to a different hospital). There was originally some particular interest in seeing how long patients whose admission had been arranged by a private consultant had waited for a hospital bed compared with those referred by NHS doctors and consultants. The number in this study referred after private consultation is small, but as can be seen from the table 3.3, there is some indication that private patients were more likely to wait less than a week than the other two groups.

Bearing in mind what has been said previously about factors that may affect how long a patient waits for admission, the differences between those referred by their GP and those whose admission was arranged by the outpatient department of a hospital, may have arisen if the patients already attending hospital as outpatients are those with the more serious conditions needing the more urgent treatment.

As stated earlier the main concern in the survey was not to collect factual data on length of waiting times for admission, but rather to find out how patients felt about having to wait for a hospital bed.

Over half (56%) of the 312 waiting list patients said that they had not been given any idea how long they might have to wait for a hospital bed to become available, but it was interesting to find that only 21 of these 176 patients (12%) found it inconvenient not knowing how long they might have to wait; to the majority it didn't really matter.

Of the 127 patients who had been told what to expect, well over half (60%) said that in fact they were admitted more or less on time; only 11% waited longer than they had expected, while the remaining 29% were actually admitted earlier.[16]

One in five of the 312 waiting list patients said that the wait between being told they were going into hospital and being admitted caused them distress or inconvenience. As can clearly be seen from the table below the longer the wait the more likely was the patient to be disturbed in some way by it, this despite the fact that one might expect those waiting the longer periods to be the patients with the less serious, less urgent, or less incapacitating conditions.

Table 3.4   Proportion of patients caused distress or inconvenience by waiting for hospital admission

Whether waiting for admission caused distress or inconvenience	Time between first being told and being admitted					All
	less than 2 weeks	2 weeks – less 1 month	1 month – less 3 months	3 months – less 6 months	6 months or longer	
	%	%	%	%	%	%
wait caused distress/ inconvenience	9	12	19	31	39	20
wait did not cause distress	91	88	81	69	61	80
Base: all who had a bed booked for first admission=100%	75	57	64	59	41	301

Nearly half (47%) of the 60 patients who were distressed or inconvenienced by waiting for hospital admission said this was because their condition was causing them pain; one in three said that their condition was in some way limiting their activities, either their work, their home or their social life, and one in six said that they were worried about what was wrong with them or about how serious their complaint was. There was no evidence to suggest that women found the wait more distressing or inconvenient than men, nor that younger people were less concerned than older patients.

It may be of interest to note that 31 of the 312 waiting list patients said that they had been given a date for admission which was subsequently changed; in 17 cases it had been the patient's decision alone to postpone admission but in 12 cases—4% of the 312 booked admissions—the hospital alone had been responsible for changing the date.

Length of notice for admission

Having waited several weeks or perhaps months for admission, a patient may then be given very little notice that the hospital is ready for them: we looked to see how much notice patients had been given of admission, and whether or not they felt this was sufficient time for them.

Twenty two of the 312 waiting list patients had been given an actual date for admission when they were originally told they had to go into hospital, but where the date of admission was not already known, between two days and a weeks notice was the most frequent practice. Ten per cent of patients were given less than 24 hours notice that the hospital was ready to admit them, but 20 of these 28

16. Fourteen patients asked for their admission to be delayed for their own convenience; this was agreed to in every case, and only one patient felt that this resulted in their waiting much longer for a bed; for the remainder, admission was put back to about the time they had wanted.

Table 3.5 How much notice patients were given that the hospital had a bed ready for them

Amount of notice	%
Less than 24 hours	10
24 hours—less than 48 hours	8
2 days—less than 1 week	39
1 week—less than 2 weeks	32
2 weeks or longer	11
Base: all who had a bed booked for first admission[1]=100%	282

1. excludes 22 patients originally given definite date for admission

patients were admitted within a week of being told they had to go into hospital; two of the 28 had however been waiting between six and 12 months for a bed.

Only seven patients said that they had not been given adequate notice of admission; representing 2% of all 312 waiting list patients. Three of these seven patients had been given less than 24 hours notice of admission and two out of these three were non-working mothers with very young children to look after, for whom sudden admission to hospital may well have caused particular problems.

3.2 Waiting for a first outpatient appointment

As with those who had been admitted to hospital as inpatients, for outpatients we were most interested in the circumstances of the first outpatient appointment that the patient had been given for the sampled condition, remembering that for many patients this first visit to hospital had taken place prior to the beginning of the three month reference period. The table below shows who first referred the patient to the hospital as an outpatient.

Table 3.6 Who referred patient to hospital for first outpatient visit

Source of referral to outpatients	%
Patient's GP, family doctor	76
Outpatient dept of another hospital	8
Referred after spell as inpatient	9
Private consultant or specialist	1
Other	6
Base: all who had an appointment for their first outpatient visit=100%	1491

Excluded from this table are the 776 men and women (34% of the total sample) whose first visit to hospital for the sampled condition was made without an appointment or who had first attended as casualty, accident or emergency cases.

As would be expected the majority of patients had been referred to the hospital initially by their own GP, with small proportions having their first outpatient appointment initiated either by an outpatient department at another hospital they had been attending, or following on from an inpatient spell. The small group of patients referred by other sources are those who reported that their first outpatient appointment was arranged by doctors other than those already specified, such as opticians, dentists, school doctors and doctors at the patient's place of work.

Only a very small proportion (1%) reported that they had been referred to hospital as an NHS patient after seeing a consultant or specialist on a private fee-paying basis. This very small number of referrals by doctors consulted privately has again made it impossible for us to compare reliably the time a 'private' patient waits for an outpatient appointment, with the time waited by patients referred under the NHS.

In looking at the length of time patients had waited for their first outpatient appointment, apart from excluding those who had attended as casualties or without an appointment, it was also decided to exclude any other patient whose first appointment had been before 1975, mainly because it seemed unlikely that they would remember the details of a visit made that long ago.

As can be seen from the table below over a quarter of the patients waited no more than seven days for their first outpatient appointment and over half the group had been seen within three weeks.

Table 3.7   How long patients who were referred to hospital as outpatients by their GPs waited for their first appointment

How long patients waited for their first appointment	Patient was referred to hospital . . .				All
	by their GP/family doctor	by out-patient dept. at another hospital	after inpatient spell	by other sources incl. private consultant/ specialist	
	cum %	cum %	cum %	cum %	cum %
7 days or less	26	43	34	29	28
8–14 days	43	60	44	41	45
15–21 days	58	67	54	56	60
22–28 days	70	69	68	70	72
over 4 weeks–5 weeks	77	73	75	75	78
over 5 weeks–6 weeks	82	78	84	78	83
over 6 weeks–3 months	93	87	99	95	94
over 3 months	100	100	100	100	100
Base: all who had an appointment for their first outpatient visit=100%	702	54	77	65	898

However one in five patients had waited over five weeks for this their first outpatient appointment. It can also be seen from the table that 60% of those who had been referred from an outpatients department at some other hospital were seen within two weeks on this first occasion, whereas only 43% of those referred by other sources had been seen that quickly.

The data also showed that patients whose first visit was to an ancillary department, for example, for physiotherapy, were more likely to have been given a first appointment within seven days than patients attending consultative outpatient departments (see table 1 Appendix III). Most patients were however, attending as consultative outpatients, and of these just under half waited more than three weeks for their first appointment; we now look at how distressing they, and patients attending ancillary departments, found waiting for this first appointment.

One in five patients who had waited longer than seven days for their first outpatient appointment said that they had minded waiting that long, representing about one in seven overall of all whose first outpatient visit was by appointment: to the majority the wait had not really mattered. As can clearly be seen from the table below the longer the wait for this first appointment the more likely was the patient to have been worried or distressed by it; less than one in ten of those who had waited between eight and 14 days for their first outpatient appointment said they minded waiting that long, compared with just under half of those whose first appointment took over six weeks to arrange.

Table 3.8   Proportion of patients who minded waiting for their first outpatient appointment

Whether minded waiting for first appointment	Time waited for first outpatient appointment					All
	8–14 days	15–21 days	22–28 days	over 4 weeks— 6 weeks	over 6 weeks	
	%	%	%	%	%	%
Patient minded waiting	7	11	20	22	44	21
Wait didn't really matter	93	89	80	78	56	79
Base=100%[1].	147	130	106	102	157	642

1. Base=all who waited more than 7 days for their first outpatient appointment

Although there was no difference between the proportion of men and the proportion of women who minded waiting for their first appointment, analysis showed that patients aged between 17 and 54 and the parents of child patients aged under 10 were more likely to have been concerned by the delay than patients of other ages.

Table 3.9   Proportion of patients in different age groups who minded waiting for their first outpatient appointment

Whether minded waiting for first appointment	Patients aged:						All men	All women
	0–9	10–16	17–34	35–54	55–64	65 and over		
	%	%	%	%	%	%	%	%
Minded waiting	22	15	27	28	14	12	21	22
Wait didn't really matter	78	85	73	72	86	88	79	78
Base=100%[1]	76	46	142	172	101	106	288	355

1. Base=all who waited more than 7 days for their first appointment.

Two main reasons emerged as to why patients minded waiting for their first outpatient appointment; both were reasons that might have been expected, but it was interesting to find that they were put forward in approximately equal numbers. Sixty nine of the 140 patients (49%) who were upset by the wait said this was because they were concerned to know what was wrong with them, or how serious their condition was. The following is typical of the answers in this category; this from a patient who waited five weeks for a first appointment . . .

"My eye was getting bad and I wanted to know what was wrong with me. I wanted to know whether it was serious or not".

Seventy four patients (53%) minded waiting because they were suffering physical pain or discomfort, or in a few cases, embarrassment from their complaint. This category included the following answers from two patients:

"My face was distorted, and I couldn't go out, I was extremely uncomfortable and I was in some pain".

"It was a bit inconvenient having a cyst on my head—it kept bleeding, and in my job I'm meeting people all the time".

A small number of patients mentioned both these reasons—the worry about knowing what was wrong, and the pain—for minding about waiting for their first appointment. A variety of other reasons, each mentioned by only a few patients, but put together accounting for 15%, were also given; these included people who were worried, not about what was wrong with them, but simply because they had not heard from the hospital; they wondered if they had been forgotten, their details lost, or whether it was their responsibility to make the appointment.

There were also a small number of patients who, because of their condition, were absent from their work; they minded waiting for an appointment because they felt the sooner they were seen, the sooner they could get back to their job, and as might have been expected, there were a very few patients who said they were either very much better by the time they got the appointment, or that there was no longer any need to see the doctor . . .

"By the time I was seen the knee had gone down—if they had seen me earlier they might have found something".

3.3 Summary

In this chapter we have looked at the length of time patients waited either for admission to hospital as an inpatient, or for their first outpatient appointment, and at the effect on the patient of any delay.

We found that over a quarter of the patients admitted to hospital from a waiting list had been admitted within two weeks of being told they would have to go into hospital, and that nearly half had been admitted within one month. Over half of those who had been told what sort of wait to expect said they had been admitted more or less on time, and over a quarter had been admitted even earlier than they thought they would be. About one in twenty of all patients given some idea of how long they might have to wait said they had been given a date for admission but that it had subsequently been changed by the hospital. A comparatively small, but nevertheless significant proportion of all 'waiting list' patients (7%) minded not being told how long they might have to wait for admission; some general idea of what to expect would obviously be appreciated by a number of patients. Overall, one in five patients were distressed or inconvenienced by the wait for admission, but among those who had waited for over three months this proportion rose steeply to one in three. The distress was generally attributed to the pain caused by the patient's condition, with only a small proportion being worried about finding out what was wrong with them. This contrasts sharply with the views expressed by outpatients where nearly half of those who were concerned at the delay in waiting for their first appointment said this was because they were concerned to find out what was wrong with them or how serious their condition was. The findings showed that the amount of notice of admission given to the patient by the hospital, even when it was very short (less than 24 hours) caused few problems for patients: only 2% said it was insufficient.

4.0   Getting to the hospital

In this chapter we look at the journeys inpatients made to hospital on the occasion when they were being admitted, and for outpatients, on the various occasions they had to attend hospital as casualty patients or by appointment.

Two areas were of particular interest: firstly we wanted to know what proportion of those who had made their own way to hospital would have preferred hospital transport to have been laid on for them and for what reasons and secondly, since it is popularly held that the hospital transport service is often unreliable and otherwise unsatisfactory, we wanted to know how patients who had been taken to or from hospital by ambulance or hospital car felt about the service.

Getting to the hospital is more likely to be a major consideration to the outpatient who has to make several visits to hospital, than to the inpatient who has just the one journey there and back; we therefore look first in this chapter at the experiences and attitudes of the outpatients we spoke to.

4.1   How outpatients got to and from the hospital

In asking outpatients how they got to and from the hospital we decided to look at all the journeys they had made for the sampled condition and not just at one visit in particular, we are therefore able to show (in table 4.1 below) the proportion of patients who *always* used hospital transport, the proportion who *always* made their own way there, and the proportion who *sometimes* used transport laid on by the hospital and on other occasions made their own arrangements: naturally anyone who only made one outpatient visit *always* used either one method or the other.

Table 4.1   How men and women outpatients got to and from the hospital

Getting back from the hospital	Getting to the hospital						All outpatients	
	Always by hospital transport		Sometimes by hospital transport		Always made own way			
	Nos	%	Nos	%	Nos	%	Nos	%
Always by hospital transport	149	7	5	*	7	*	161	7
Sometimes by hospital transport	6	*	72	3	5	*	83	4
Always made own way	31	1	31	1	1944	86	2006	89
All outpatients[1]	186	8	108	5	1956	87	2250	100

1. excludes eight patients who made only one outpatient visit to hospital which resulted in their being admitted: two were taken to hospital by ambulance, six made their own way there.

The great majority of patients, as would be expected, had always made their own way both to and from the hospital; less than one in ten patients had always been taken and brought back by transport laid on by the hospital, and indeed only 306 patients (14%) had any experience of using hospital transport at all.

Further analysis clearly showed that the older patients, those aged 65 and over, were far more likely to have had hospital transport arranged to take them to and from the hospital than younger men and women.

Table 4.2   How men and women in different age groups got to and from the hospital

Transport to and from the hospital	Men and women aged						All
	0–9	10–16	17–34	35–54	55–64	65 & over	
	%	%	%	%	%	%	%
Always by hospital transport	3	1	2	2	7	24	6
Sometimes used hospital transport	6	8	7	8	5	12	8
Always made own way	91	91	91	90	88	64	86
Base: all outpatients=100%	296	229	505	531	314	392	2267

Less than one in twenty patients aged under 65 had always had hospital transport arranged to take them to and from the hospital, compared with one in four of those aged 65 and over. The elderly were also more likely than younger outpatients to have used hospital transport on only some occasions, so that overall one in three patients aged 65 and over had on at least one occasion used hospital transport to get either to or from the hospital compared with only about one in ten patients aged under 65.

It was not possible to see whether the distance to the hospital and the time the journey took affected the likelihood of a patient being given hospital transport, since, as we shall see later in this section, information on journey time to the hospital for patients travelling by ambulance or hospital car included the time taken to collect other patients on the way to the hospital.

Those who made their own way to or from the hospital

This section looks at the methods of transport used to get to and from the hospital by patients who, *on any occasion,* made their own way either there or back. Patients who made their own way to and from the hospital on more than one occasion were asked about their usual arrangements and about how long it usually took them to make the journey. In this discussion we talk therefore about patients' usual arrangements and experiences, but are of course including patients with only one visit to hospital, and those who made their own way there or back on just one occasion.

Most of those who made their own way to or from the hospital went by private transport, indeed overall nearly half (48%) of the patients usually went by private car (or motorcycle) to and from the hospital—see table 4.3 below.

Just under a third had a journey which involved using public transport in both directions and just under one in ten patients usually walked all the way there and back. A very small number of patients either paid for a hire car or a taxi to take

Table 4.3 Method of transport used by those patients who made their own way to, and/or from the hospital on at least one occasion

Getting back from the hospital	Getting to the hospital													All who made own way back from hospital[1]	
	Walked all the way		Private car or m/cycle		Hired car or taxi		Bus, train, or tube		Firm's car		Other				
	Nos	%	Nos	%	Nos	%	Nos	%	Nos	%	Nos	%		Nos	%
Walked all the way	178=8%		7		2		8		—		—			194	9%
Private car or m/cycle	1		1090=48%		3		59		1		9			1151	51%
Hired car or taxi	7		17		38=2%		27		—		—			81	4%
Bus, train, tube	7		77		30		623=27%		2		8			688	30%
Firm's car	—		5		—		—		19=1%		—			19	1%
Other	—		—		—		6		—		28=1%			28	1%
All who made their own way to hospital[1]	201=9%		1157=51%		64=3%		667=29%		22=1%		35=2%			2267	100%

Base: all outpatients

1. Numbers may add to more than sum of columns or rows since, except for people who walked all the way, all methods of transport used were recorded.

them to or from the hospital, or were taken to hospital by a car belonging to the firm where they worked.

The table below (table 4.4) shows how long it usually took patients who made their own way to *and* from the hospital to get there and back, and we were somewhat surprised to find that for over half this group of patients the journey usually took less than about 15 minutes each way. However for one in ten patients it usually took about an hour or longer to get to the hospital and then the same back again, and four patients, included in this group, told us that it usually took them at least two hours each way.

Table 4.4   Time taken to get to and from hospital by all outpatients who made their own way there *and* their own way back on at least one occasion

Time usually taken to get back from hospital	Time usually taken to get to the hospital				Total	
	about 15 mins or less	about 30 mins	about 45 mins	about 1 hour or more		
	Nos %	Nos %	Nos %	Nos %	Nos	%
about 15 mins or less	1183=58%	13	5	5	1206	59%
about 30 mins	55	375=18%	8	3	441	22%
about 45 mins	9	17	156=8%	8	190	9%
about 1 hour or more	9	10	9	180=9%	208	10%
Total	1256=61%	415=20%	178=9%	196=10%	2045=	100%

Base: all who made their own way to *and* from hospital on at least one occasion=2045=100%

Although we cannot tell whether patients who lived further from the hospital were more, or even less likely, to be provided with hospital transport, than those who lived relatively close to the hospital, we were able to see whether patients being taken by ambulance or hospital car spent longer getting to the hospital (which includes the time taken to collect other patients) than those who made their own way there.

The analysis showed that a much greater proportion of those who used hospital transport spent about three quarters of an hour or longer getting to or from the hospital compared to those who made their own arrangements. Well over half of the patients making their own way there or back took less than about 15 minutes to get to the hopsital, and the same to get back home again; this compared with only about one third of those who were taken by ambulance or hospital car.

Table 4.5   Time taken to get to and from the hospital by patients who used hospital transport and by those who made their own way

Time usually taken:	Getting to the hospital:		Getting back from the hospital:	
	used hospital transport[1]	made own way	used hospital transport	made own way
	%	%	%	%
about 15 mins or less	33	61	33	60
about 30 mins	30	20	33	21
about 45 mins	16	9	17	9
about 1 hour or more	21	10	17	10
Base: all using method of transport on at least one occasion=100%	215	2071	239	2086

1. excludes those whose only use of hospital transport was as emergency or accident case

How patients felt about the time it took to get to or from hospital by ambulance, and whether they minded having to collect or drop off other patients is discussed later in this chapter. However when we look at the people who said they would have preferred to have had hospital transport laid on for them rather than having to make their own way, we shall look to see whether the time it took to get to or from hospital had any relationship to this expressed preference.

Of the 2074 men and women who made their own way to hospital on at least one occasion 95 (5%) said they would have preferred hospital transport to have been provided to get them there, and of the 2086 people who had made their own way back from hospital, 94 (5%) said they would have preferred hospital transport back. Of course many patients expressed a preference for hospital transport both there and back, so that by further analysis we found 69 patients who would have liked the hospital to have arranged transport both to *and* from the hospital for them, 26 patients who would have liked hospital transport to take them there, and a further 25 patients who would have liked an ambulance or hospital car to take them home. If all 116 patients had been given hospital transport, then the proportion being taken either to and/or from hospital by ambulance or hospital car on at least one occasion would have increased by just 5%.

We have already seen that elderly patients, those aged 65 and over, were more likely to have been given hospital transport to get to or from the hospital on at least one occasion, than younger patients. Our analysis (table 4.6 below) showed clearly that elderly patients who had made their own way to or from the hospital were no more likely to have said that they would have preferred hospital transport to have been laid on for them than younger patients, suggesting that the demand from the elderly, who are most likely to want or need hospital transport, is largely being met.

Table 4.6 Proportions of men and women in different age groups who would have preferred the hospital to have laid on transport to take them to or from the hospital

Patients' preference for hospital transport	Getting to the hospital:							Getting back from the hospital:						
	Men and women aged:				All men	All women	Men & women	Men and women aged:				All men	All women	Men & women
	0–16	17–54	55–64	65 & over				0–16	17–54	55–64	65 & over			
	%	%	%	%	%	%	%	%	%	%	%	%	%	%
Would have preferred hospital transport	5	4	4	7	4	5	5	4	4	5	5	4	5	5
Hospital transport not necessary	95	96	96	93	96	95	95	96	96	95	95	96	95	95
Base=100%[1]	502	994	290	288	1076	998	2074	504	1002	289	291	1084	1002	2086

1. Base=all who made their own way to or from the hospital on at least one occasion.

Table 4.7 Proportions of those whose journey to or from hospital took about an hour or longer who would have preferred hospital transport to have been laid on for them

Patients' preference for hospital transport	Journey to hospital usually took:				Journey back from hospital usually took:			
	about 15 mins or less	about 30 mins	about 45 mins	about 1 hour or more	about 15 mins or less	about 30 mins	about 45 mins	about 1 hour or more
	%	%	%	%	%	%	%	%
Preferred hospital transport	2	5	8	20	2	4	8	20
Not necessary	98	95	92	80	98	96	92	80
Base=100%[1]	1273	420	179	199	1237	446	190	213

1. Base=all who made their own way to or from the hospital on at least one occasion.

However as we had suspected, the time it took the patients to get to or from the hospital affected the likelihood of their preferring hospital transport: only 3% of those whose journey to hospital usually took no more than about 45 minutes said they would have preferred hospital transport to have been laid on compared with 20% of those who had a journey of about an hour or longer.

When asked why they would have preferred hospital transport, patients gave answers which could be classified into four main groups. The most frequently mentioned reason, as can be seen from the table below, was that the form of transport used (and this includes walking) affected their condition; smokey buses and trains affected a patient with asthma, and some people who had breathing difficulties found walking a problem. A large proportion of patients said they found public transport inconvenient, it was, for example, infrequent, or the journey involved changing buses or trains. The expense involved in getting themselves to hospital, not only on public transport, but also the cost of petrol, or taxi fares, was mentioned, not as frequently as the two reasons given above, but nevertheless by a considerable proportion of patients. Finally about one in five patients who would have preferred hospital transport said it was because they felt it was inconvenient for other people, such as husbands, wives or neighbours, to have to take them to hospital, and then perhaps wait to bring them home again.

Table 4.8 **Reasons for patients preferring hospital transport to have been provided**

Reasons for patients preferring hospital transport to have been provided	Patients who would have preferred hospital transport:	
	to have taken them to hospital	to have brought them back from hospital
	%	%
Other forms of transport affect patient's health	47	50
Public transport is inconvenient	40	41
Expense of other types of transport	24	14
Inconvenience caused to friends, relatives etc	21	18
Other reasons	14	12
Base: all who would have preferred hospital transport=100%	95	92

The group of various other reasons which were each mentioned by only a few patients, included the comments from three patients who said that they would have felt safer and more reassured in an ambulance, in case they were taken ill on the journey, and from another two who would have preferred transport home as they found their treatment at the hospital so exhausting.

The data suggest therefore, that although we have found that patients with long journeys to hospital were more likely to have preferred hospital transport to have been laid on for them than those who only took a short time to get there, it is not solely the distance that the patient lives from the hospital that affects demand, but also the complexity or inconvenience of the journey. So, even though the journey may take longer by ambulance, which on our evidence, is likely, the patient may nevertheless prefer it to making his own way there because it avoids the difficulties in using public transport.

Those who were taken to, or brought back from hospital by ambulance or hospital car

We have already seen (table 4.1) that a total of 306 patients had some experience of travelling by hospital car or ambulance.

Of the patients who were taken to hospital by ambulance or hospital car, 76 (3% of the total outpatient sample) had used hospital transport to get to the hospital on only one occasion, when they were being taken as emergency or accident cases; the transport to the hospital had not been laid on by prior arrangement for them as it had for the other 218 patients. One in three of these non-emergency patients said that their transport had first been arranged by their own family doctor, in nearly all other cases the hospital had first made the arrangements.

The table below shows what transport was laid on by the hospital to take patients to and from their appointments, and, not surprisingly the analysis showed that while only 4% of patients attending hospital by appointment travelled to the hospital in stretcher ambulances, 79% of those who had been taken as emergency or casualty patients had been taken to hospital in a stretcher ambulance. The majority of patients using hospital transport either to or from the hospital had usually been taken in a wheelchair ambulance.

Table 4.9   **Transport usually provided to take patients to and from the hospital**

Hospital transport usually used:	Getting to the hospital		Returning from the hospital
	'Accident/ emergency cases'[1]	'Outpatients'	
	%	%	%
Ambulance: stretcher	79	4	7
sitting/wheelchair	21	81	79
Hospital car	—	15	14
Base: all using hospital transport=100%	76	218	241

1. Accident/emergency cases: those who only ever went to hospital by ambulance as accident or emergency cases.

Waiting for the ambulance or car to go to hospital

Two out of three patients provided with transport to the hospital for outpatient appointments said they were usually given a specific time when the ambulance or hospital car would pick them up. Twenty of the 68 patients (29%) who were not told when to expect the ambulance said they found this inconvenient, but to the rest it had not really mattered. The majority of those who had been told when to expect the ambulance said that it usually came at about the time it was supposed to, however 29 out of 148 (20%) said that it was generally not reliable. Not surprisingly more people said the transport was usually late (15 patients) than said it was usually early (8 patients). However, only four patients—less than 2% of all using hospital transport to get to the hospital—said that this mattered to them.

Perhaps the most extreme case of transport being late, is when it fails to arrive completely: three per cent of all the outpatients we spoke to said that on at least one occasion the transport that had been arranged for them had failed to pick them up. Fortunately in most cases (40 out of the 64) this had happened only once, although six patients each reported its happening to them on four separate occasions. None of these patients had, on any occasion, been warned in advance that the ambulance or car would not be able to pick them up so that they could make other arrangements to get to the hospital. Indeed 40 of these 64 patients said that they had missed their appointment completely on at least one occasion because the transport had failed to pick them up. Not only were these patients not warned beforehand that the transport would not be coming, but nearly half said they had never at any point been given any explanation as to what had happened. Although the times when patients cannot be picked up can only represent a small proportion of the total number of calls made by ambulances and hospital cars, on the occasions when it does happen it must, if nothing else, be inconvenient to the patient waiting to be collected. While it may not always be possible to get in touch with the patient at home to warn them of what is happening, some explanation ought to be given at a later stage.

Hospital transport after treatment

Patients being taken home from hospital by ambulance or hospital car may find that they have to wait for transport after they have finished being seen by the doctor either because the transport is not already laid on and special arrangements have then to be made for them to be taken home, (this is especially likely if the patient is new to the outpatient clinic, or attended as a casualty or accident case), or because several patients are to travel in the same ambulance or car, and everyone must wait until the last patient has been seen. Nearly all (90%) the patients who had been given hospital transport home, usually knew when they arrived at the hospital that they would be given transport back home. Only 25 of the 244 patients taken back by ambulance or hospital car had to have special arrangements made while they were there; too few for us to be able to tell whether they waited longer for transport home than those whose transport was already laid on.

The table below shows that nearly two thirds of these patients usually waited no more than about 30 minutes for transport to take them home after their treatment, but that one in four usually waited about an hour or even longer.

Table 4.10 How long patients usually waited after they had finished being seen before the ambulance or car left to take them home

Time patient waited for transport home	%
about 15 minutes or less	33
about 30 minutes	29
about 45 minues	13
about an hour or longer	25
Base: all returning by hospital transport=100%	239

Overall just over one in four of those patients who waited about 30 minutes or longer for the ambulance or car to take them back from the hospital said they found the wait inconvenient or distressing, although this proportion varied considerably depending on how long the wait was. Only one in ten of those who waited about 30 minutes found it distressing, compared to one in four of those who usually waited about three quarters of an hour, and one in two of those who waited about an hour or longer.

Although the numbers are comparatively small there was a clear indication that waiting around for the ambulance was far more likely to be inconvenient or distressing to younger patients than to those aged 65 or over; there was however no difference between the reactions of men and women.

Table 4.11 Proportions of men and women in different age groups who found waiting more than about 15 minutes for an ambulance inconvenient or distressing

Patients' attitudes to waiting for transport home	Men and women aged:		All men	All women	All men and women
	0–64	65 and over			
	%	%	%	%	%
Wait was inconvenient/ distressing	45	14	26	29	28
Didn't really matter	55	86	74	71	72
Base=100%[1]	71	88	70	89	159

1. Base=all who usually waited more than about 15 mins for an ambulance home

Overall 46 patients found waiting for an ambulance or hospital car to collect them or take them home either inconvenient or distressing: this represents 15% of those in the sample who had experience of using hospital transport.

Time taken to get to and from hospital

The table below shows how long it took patients using hospital transport to get to and from the hospital, and it can be seen that most patients had a comparatively short journey, despite the fact that as we shall later see, most patients had to collect or drop off other patients on their way to or from the hospital.

Table 4.12 Time taken to get to and from the hospital for patients travelling by ambulance or hospital car

Journey usually took . . .	Getting to the hospital	Returning from the hospital
	%	%
about 15 minutes or less	32	33
about 30 minutes	30	33
about 45 minutes	16	17
about 1 hour or longer	22	17
Base: all travelling by ambulance or hospital car=100%	215[1]	239

1. excludes those who only used hospital transport to get to hospital as casualty or emergency patients.

42

Although well over half the patients using hospital transport to get to or from the hospital usually had a journey of no more than about 30 minutes, nearly one in five (19%) of those using hospital transport to get there, and a similar proportion (16%) of those travelling back by ambulance or hospital car, said that on at least one occasion the journey had taken much longer than they thought it would. However further analysis showed that this was more likely to have happened where the patient usually had a journey to or from the hospital of about an hour or longer, than where their journey was a comparatively short one. Although considerable numbers of patients did experience longer journeys than they had expected, not all were inconvenienced or distressed by it: only 12 of the 42 patients whose journey to hospital had been longer than they had expected, said that they had found this inconvenient or distressing. These 12 patients plus a further eight said they also found the longer journey back distressing, so that in all 20 of the 306 patients (7%) who had used hospital transport either to get to or from the hospital, had been distressed or inconvenienced by a journey which had taken longer than they thought it would.

The journey to or from hospital

We have already seen that only a small proportion of patients said that the ambulance or hospital car was usually late in collecting them to take them to hospital; that this proportion is small is particularly reassuring when it is appreciated that in most cases an ambulance will, on the same journey, have to collect a number of patients to take to hospital together. We found only ten patients who usually travelled to hospital alone; the other 208 (95%) usually went in the ambulance or car with other patients.

If the ambulance does have to pick up a number of patients, then for those collected early on, the journey to hospital may not be by the most direct route. Of the 218 patients taken for outpatient appointments by ambulance or hospital car, 186 (85%) said they usually called for other patients on the way to the hospital, and 99 (45%) said that this meant the ambulance (or car) had to go out of its way. However not nearly as many patients as one might expect found this an unsatisfactory arrangement: indeed there were slightly more who quite enjoyed the trip around (57 patients) than who would have preferred to have gone straight to the hospital (42 patients). Although the numbers involved were rather small, there was some indication that the older patients, aged 65 and over, were more likely to have enjoyed the trip around than younger patients, the proportions were 65% and 49% respectively.

Similarly on the journey back from hospital a number of patients may travel together in the same ambulance or car, which may mean that for any one patient the journey home may not be by the most direct route.

Of the 244 patients who used hospital transport to get home, 71 (29%) said that because other patients had to be dropped off they personally were taken out of their way; all other patients had either travelled alone, were the first to be dropped off, or found that the other patients travelling with them lived more or less on their way home. Those who were taken out of their way were almost equally divided into those who quite enjoyed the trip around (55%) and those who would have preferred to have been taken straight back (45%, or 13% of all using hospital transport to get home).

If we consider all 306 patients who had on any occasion been taken to hospital or brought back home again by ambulance or hospital car, we find that 53 patients (17%) were taken out of their way both on the journey to hospital and again on the journey back, that 21 of these 53 patients would have preferred to have gone straight there and straight back, and that 28 said they enjoyed the trip around on the way to and back from the hospital. In all 53 patients (17%) would have preferred not to have been taken out of their way either on their journey to or back from hospital.

Comfort on the journey

Very few patients had any complaints about the comfort of the ambulance or hospital car they had travelled in either to or from the hospital, and of the 23 who had usually found the journey uncomfortable ten felt that nothing could have been done to improve the situation. Seven of the 13 patients who did offer suggestions felt that the suspension in the ambulances could have been improved, three patients said their ambulances were too crowded, and two mothers would have liked special seats for babies so that they did not have their children sitting on their laps for the whole journey.

4.2 How inpatients got to the hospital

Emergency admissions

Some 45% of inpatients were admitted as emergencies, two thirds being taken to hospital by ambulance, the rest making their own way there or being taken by friends or relatives. About 20% of those admitted as emergencies were unconscious at the time, or had no awareness of the time it had taken either for the ambulance to arrive or of the time taken to get to hospital. However 15 of the 167 emergency patients who were aware of time complained that they had too long to wait before the ambulance arrived. The majority of emergency patients who were able to make an estimate, said it had taken about 15 minutes for the ambulance to get to the hospital (72%) and a further 18% said it had taken about half an hour.

Non-emergency admissions

Only 49 (10%) non-emergency admissions used hospital transport. Of these 49, 28 patients had been told when they would be called for, and three quarters of them said the ambulance arrived at about the expected time; two inpatients complained that the ambulance arriving late had mattered to them. The other 21 patients had not been told when to expect the ambulance, and here again, two patients said they would have found it more convenient had they been given an expected arrival time. Thus four of the 49 non-emergency patients using hospital transport were dissatisfied with the arrangements.

Of the 405 non-emergency patients who had made their own way to hospital or had been taken by friends or relatives, only a small proportion (4%) would have preferred the hospital to have arranged for either an ambulance or a hospital car to take them there; the overwhelming majority felt that it had not really been necessary. Six of these 18 patients would have preferred hospital transport because the journey to hospital was long, complicated, or awkward, but a further three patients said that because of their condition they found it particularly uncomfortable or painful travelling on buses or trains. Three people said that the pain or discomfort they would have suffered travelling by public transport made them take a taxi to the hospital; one of these three spontaneously mentioned that she would have willingly paid for hospital transport. Two women said it had been inconvenient because their husbands had taken time off work to take them to hospital, and here again, one mentioned her willingness to pay for hospital transport. Only one of the 18 patients who would have preferred hospital transport gave as the reason the cost to themselves of using public transport.

Comfort on the journey to hospital by ambulance

Of the total of 276 patients who were taken to hospital by ambulance or hospital car, 15 found their journey, bearing in mind their condition, uncomfortable, although it should be noted that 38 of the emergency cases were unconscious during their journey to hospital and so were unable to comment. However, seven of the 15 patients felt that nothing could have been done to make the journey more comfortable, and a further two could offer no suggestions for improvements. The suggestions that were made were, however, all different; the first two comments came from 'stretcher' patients:

—*being 'loaded' into the ambulance feet first might have helped prevent travel sickness;*

—*being propped up with pillows on the stretcher would have been more comfortable and being strapped in more securely would have minimised movement.*

A patient travelling by hospital car would have preferred fewer passengers to have been carried at the same time, and a man with a leg injury felt a stretcher ambulance would have been more suitable, and would have made it unnecessary for him to walk out to the ambulance, and then from the ambulance into the hospital. Finally one man would have preferred a newer and more comfortable ambulance; he was told that for infectious cases, the old ambulance was used as it had to be fumigated afterwards!

4.3 Summary

From the results of our survey there seems to be some dissatisfaction, both from patients who made their own way to the hospital, and who would have preferred hospital transport to have been laid on, and from those actually travelling to or from the hospital by ambulance or hospital car.

The overwhelming majority of both outpatients and non-emergency inpatients made their own way to hospital, and 5% of each of these groups said they would have preferred the hospital to have laid on transport to get them there. The demand for hospital transport would seem therefore largely to have been met, even among the elderly: elderly men and women making their own way to hospital for outpatient appointments were no more likely to have preferred hospital transport than younger patients. Hospital transport would have been preferred by those with long journeys and by those who found using public transport difficult.

The largest source of dissatisfaction with the hospital transport service concerned the time outpatients had to wait after they had finished being seen before the ambulance or car left to take them home: one in four patients returning by hospital transport said they usually waited an hour or longer, and one in four of all who waited about 30 minutes or longer said they found having to wait that long inconvenient or distressing. Small proportions of patients said that the ambulance usually arrived late to pick them up from home and take them to the hospital or that they found this inconvenient although about 7% of all using hospital transport to get to the hospital for outpatient appointments found it inconvenient not being given some idea of when to expect the ambulance or car.

Only 2% of all outpatients said that they had ever missed an appointment because an ambulance had failed to pick them up, but we feel that it is rather unfortunate that only half the patients who had been left without an ambulance had ever been given an explanation as to why it had failed to arrive.

5.0   Facilities provided for patients

This chapter looks at the provision and demand for certain facilities and amenities at the hospital, which while they may not all be essential, may make a visit to outpatients or a stay in hospital as an inpatient pass more pleasantly.

For inpatients, before discussing what facilities were provided for patients in the ward and in the hospital, patients' satisfaction with them, and the demand for facilities not available, we describe briefly the ward or room that the patient was in during their spell in hospital; we look at its size, and at how full it was while the patient was there.

In the chapter that follows this, which is only concerned with inpatients, various aspects of life as an inpatient in hospital, ward routine, meals, visiting arrangements and so on are considered. We also discuss patients' views on the size of the ward they were in, the advantages and disadvantages of being in a single room or a large ward, and look at what sort of ward patients said they would prefer to be in given the choice.

The size of the ward, the day-to-day living arrangements, and the provision of facilities such as a dayroom, a radio, or a television, are all aspects of a stay in hospital which can have a considerable impact on how favourably a patient remembers the time spent there.

5.1   Facilities for hospital inpatients

A total of 699 patients aged 14 and over were asked about the facilities and conditions in the hospital ward or room that they were in.[17]

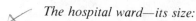

The hospital ward—its size:

Only 38 patients (6%) had spent their entire stay in hospital in a single room, although a further 12% had been in a room on their own for at least some of the time; the remaining 576 patients (82%) had been in a ward or a small room with other patients throughout their stay. As table 5.1 below shows, a slightly greater proportion of women spent at least some of their time in hospital in a room on their own, compared to the proportion of men.

Eight patients reported that they had paid for an amenity bed while they were in hospital on this occasion, but only two of these eight had been in a single room, the other six had been in a small side ward with other patients.

More than half of the 699 patients aged 14 and over had spent at least some of their time with other patients in small rooms or wards with no more than ten

---

17. Where the patient was a child aged under 14, the child's parent was asked a separate series of questions more appropriate to the conditions in a children's ward; the answers to these are reported on separately in chapter 12.

beds, nearly one in five had been in a larger ward with between 16 and 25 beds and less than one in ten had been in a ward with more than 25 beds. Not only were women more likely to have spent at least part of their stay in hospital in a single room, but as can be seen from table 5.2 below, women, and particularly maternity patients, were also more likely to have been in a small room than men; less than half of the adult men patients spoken to had been in a ward with up to ten patients compared with over three quarters of maternity patients and well over half of the other female non-maternity patients.

Table 5.1 Proportions of men and women who spent some or all of their stay in hospital in a room on their own

During their stay in hospital, patient was ...	Men	Women	Men and Women
	%	%	%
in a room on own—all of the time	3	6	6
—part of the time	10	14	12
always with other patients	87	80	82
Base: all inpatients aged 14 & over=100%	242	457	699

Table 5.2 Proportions of men and women in hospital wards of different sizes

No. of beds in ward or part of ward	Men	Women maternity patients	non-maternity patients	Men and Women
	%	%	%	%
in a single room all the time	3	5	7	5
2–4 beds	20	37	26	26
5–10 beds	25	41	26	28
11–15 beds	16	9	14	14
16–25 beds	26	6	18	19
more than 25 beds	10	2	9	8
Base: all inpatients aged 14 and over=100%	242	97	359	698

However, one in ten of those who had been in a room or ward with other patients for at least some of the time said that half or less than half the beds in their ward or in their part of the ward were occupied, and there was some evidence to suggest that it was the larger wards that were full—table 5.3. below.

Table 5.3 Proportions of beds that were occupied in hospital wards of different sizes

Proportion of beds that were occupied	No. of beds in ward, or part of ward					All
	Up to 4	5–10	11–15	16–25	over 25	
	%	%	%	%	%	%
all or nearly all	89	87	94	95	98	91
about half	8	8	6	4	2	7
less than half	3	5	—	1	—	2
Base=100%	177	193	98	132	58	658

Amenities in the hospital for patients

All patients aged 14 and over were asked about the provision of a number of amenities for patients in the hospital generally and in the ward or room they were in, and as can be seen from the table below the level of provision was generally very high.

Table 5.4   Provision of various amenities for patients in hospital

Provision of amenity	Amenity				
	Dayroom/ restroom	TV	Radio/ earphones	Telephone	Shop or ward trolley service
	%	%	%	%	%
Provided	76	90	78	94	90
Not provided	19	8	21	3	9
Patient didn't know	5	2	1	3	1
Base: all inpatients aged 14 and over=100%	699	699	699	699	699

Of the 628 patients who were able to watch television while they were in hospital, 194 (31%) had a TV set in their ward or in the room they were in, and remarkably only 12 patients said they were sometimes disturbed by it being on.

We were somewhat surprised to find that the provision of hospital radios and earphones was not more extensive, but although 3% of those without a hospital radio had taken their own radio into hospital with them, there remained 18% of adult patients who were without any radio at all. Where earphones or a radio were provided they were not always used, neither did they always work satisfactorily. Of the 546 patients provided with a radio or earphones, 29% said they had not used them, and 16% that they did not work properly. As we then found that over a third of those patients with radios that had been used and that had worked all right, were not generally able to get the radio stations they wanted to listen to, there does seem to be room for some improvement in this service. However, as can be seen from the table that follows, a large proportion (77%) of those who were without any radio were not bothered by this.

Telephones: In addition to asking whether patients were able to make telephone calls out from the hospital, we also asked whether, more unusually, they were able to take incoming calls. Where a considerable number of patients in a ward are bedfast it is probably inconvenient for the staff to arrange for patients to take incoming calls, and it may also be irritating to other patients to have a phone ringing, or, if they are mobile, to feel they have to take messages. Whereas almost all patients said they could make outgoing telephone calls, only a quarter were able also to take incoming calls, but of these 174 patients only five (3%) objected to this being possible. Over two thirds were positively in favour and pleased that it was possible, while the remaining 29% did not mind one way or the other.

Again nearly all the patients we spoke to were able to buy newspapers, magazines, sweets and cigarettes, or toilet articles while they were in hospital either from a hospital shop (40%) or more frequently from a mobile trolley service that visited the wards (84%).

Although the level of provision of amenities was in every case high, nevertheless we have looked at the demand for such facilities where they were not available. As can be seen from the table below, although the majority of patients were not bothered by the lack of certain amenities, there was nevertheless in every case a substantial proportion who would have found their provision useful.

Table 5.5   Proportions of patients who would have liked the provision of certain amenities which were not available to them while they were in hospital

Patients' attitudes to provision of amenity	Amenity			
	Dayroom/ restroom	Radio	Telephone (for out- going calls)	Shop or ward trolley service
	%	%	Nos.	%
Patient would have liked facility	38	23	[4]	46
Was not really bothered	62	77	[18]	54
Base: all inpatients aged 14 and over for whom facility was not available=100%	131	127	22	59

There was least demand for a telephone that patients could use to make out-going calls, with four of the 22 patients who had not had access to a phone saying they would have liked to have been able to make calls out. The provision of a dayroom or rest room, where patients could go and sit, and a hospital shop or a ward trolley service, were more in demand; nearly half the patients who had neither a shop nor a trolley service would have found such a provision useful, and over a third of the patients who had been in hospital without a dayroom would have liked somewhere to sit, other than the ward, when they were out of bed. Although the numbers were small, it was clear from further analysis that the real demand for a dayroom came from the male patients; over half (25 out of 44) of the men would have liked such a room to have been available, compared with just over a quarter (25 out of 87) of the women.[18]

The provisions that we have considered so far have been those which could be described as social amenities, rather than facilities for personal care. The provision of adequate washing, bathing and toilet facilities, which we now go on to look at, most patients would probably agree, is more important than the provision of televisions or dayrooms.

Most adult patients when asked, said they found the washing and bathing facilities and the toilets in the hospital satisfactory. But although overall about 80% of patients were satisfied with these facilities, there was, as can be seen from the table below, considerably more dissatisfaction from women generally and in particular from maternity patients than from men: two out of every five maternity patients found the washing or bathing facilities unsatisfactory and one in four found the toilets unsatisfactory.

18. We looked to see whether the demand for a dayroom came from men who were not allowed to smoke in their own room or ward, but found no evidence to support this.

Table 5.6 Proportions of men and women inpatients who found the washing and bathing facilities and the toilet facilities satisfactory

Facilities were:	Washing and bathing facilities				Toilet (W.C.) facilities			
	Men	Women		Men and Women	Men	Women		Men and Women
		maternity patients	non-maternity patients			maternity patients	non-maternity patients	
	%	%	%	%	%	%	%	%
Satisfactory	85	59	78	78	86	75	80	82
Unsatisfactory	12	41	19	19	11	25	16	15
Not used	3	—	3	3	3	—	3	3
Base: all inpatients aged 14 & over=100%	242	97	360	699	242	97	363	699

The main complaint about the washing and bathing facilities was that there were an inadequate number of baths; nearly two thirds of those dissatisfied with the bathing arrangements mentioned this. Maternity patients may want and need to take more frequent baths than patients in hospital for other conditions, and although the numbers were small, it was clear that the inadequate number of baths and showers was of particular concern to them. A much smaller proportion of patients (about one in three) thought there were too few washbasins for the number of patients that needed to use them, and about one in eight patients felt they did not have enough privacy when washing or bathing. In a later chapter we look in more detail at various situations where patients may have felt they had inadequate privacy, but here, although the numbers involved were small, there was some evidence to suggest that women were more likely than men to have felt they had insufficient privacy when washing or bathing.

Table 5.7   Reasons for patients finding the washing or bathing facilities in hospital unsatisfactory

Reasons for facilities being unsatisfactory	%
Not enough baths	64
Not enough washbasins	30
Not enough showers	10
Lack of privacy	13
Washbasins/baths not kept clean	10
One or more washbasins/baths/showers not working	7
Other reasons	24
Base: all who found the washing or bathing facilities in hospital unsatisfactory=100%	136

Small numbers of patients complained that the baths or basins were not kept clean, or that they were out of order, and the most common complaints included in the group of other infrequently mentioned reasons were that the bathrooms were cold to stand around in, and very cramped. A small number of patients were unhappy at bowls of water being brought to them to wash their face and hands in bed; they felt they were capable of going to the bathroom for a *"proper wash"*.

Toilet facilities

There were really only two major complaints about the toilet facilities: there were not enough toilets, mentioned by two thirds of those dissatisfied, and they were always dirty, mentioned by one in four—a significantly higher proportion than we found complaining of dirty washbasins or baths. Less than 5% of those dissatisfied said this was because the toilets were often not working, and again small numbers of patients mentioned that the toilets were cold or draughty, very cramped, or a long way from the ward or room they were in. There were a number of complaints about the poor quality and hardness of the toilet paper provided, but hardly anyone mentioned that they had been upset because there were not locks on the cubicle doors.

We also looked to see whether patients in larger wards were more likely to have been dissatisfied with the washing, bathing and toilet facilities, and in particular whether they were more likely than patients in small wards to have found the level of provision inadequate (see tables 2 and 3 in Appendix III).

There was no evidence that patients in larger wards were generally more likely to have found the washing and bathing facilities unsatisfactory, although it was clear from the analysis that patients in the very largest wards, those with more than 25 beds, were considerably less satisfied with the toilets (WC's) provided than patients who were in smaller wards: 63% of those in wards for more than 25 patients were dissatisfied compared with over 80% of those in smaller wards. However the reasons why patients in larger wards were dissatisfied, and in particular the number of complaints about inadequate provision of toilets, showed the same distribution as those given by patients in smaller wards.

At this point, while considering patients' satisfaction with toilet facilities, it is worth noting that of the 463 adult patients who, at some time during their stay in hospital had had to use a bedpan or a bottle because they were unable to get out of bed to go to the toilet, 90% said they never had any difficulty in getting a bedpan or bottle when they wanted it. A similarly high proportion said it was always taken away promptly after use; 4% said they were sometimes left with it longer during the night, and 6% thought the staff were always slow in removing it.

5.2   Facilities for hospital outpatients and those who accompanied them

We decided to restrict ourselves to asking patients about the facilities and amenities that had been provided for patients and for those who accompanied them in just one department visited while at the hospital. This was defined as the department or clinic they first went to on their last (most recent) visit to the hospital. Analysis showed however that over three quarters (77%) of patients had on their last visit only been to just the one department, they had not been sent on to any other department, for example, for X-rays or blood tests in the course of this last visit.

As we have already said many patients simply regarded themselves as having visited *"the outpatients"*, but by asking what treatment they had received or what they had gone there for, it was possible to identify the specialist clinics that some patients had attended; we suspect however that the proportion shown in table 5.8 below as attending the outpatient clinic is still an overestimate.

The first concern in asking about the conditions and facilities in the department visited, was to find out how accessible it was.

The data show that 95% of patients when they first went to this particular clinic said they had no trouble in finding it, nor if it was not on the ground floor was there generally any difficulty in getting to the department. Nearly three quarters of the patients who had to go up or down to another floor in the hospital said a lift was provided for use by patients, and only four of the 74 patients who had to use the stairs had any difficulty.

Although the provision of amenities such as refreshment bars, magazines and public telephones are no doubt useful and may make the time spent at the hospital pass more pleasantly, the provision of an adequate number of

Table 5.8 Department or clinic that patients first went to on their last (most recent) visit to hospital

Department or Clinic attended	Nos.	%
Outpatients department	1000	44
Casualty	504	22
Ophthalmic or dental clinic	118	5
X-ray department	113	5
Physiotherapy	68	3
Orthopaedic clinic	56	2
Gynaecology	48	2
Ear, nose and throat clinic	43	2
Paediatric department	28	1
Other departments and clinics[1]	287	13
Base: all outpatients=100%	2265	100

1. Includes radiotherapy, psychiatric, and diabetic clinics. No single department included in this group was attended by more than 2% of patients.

comfortable seats in the waiting area would probably be a more important priority to patients waiting for treatment.

Most patients (87%) said that there were usually enough seats provided for everyone who was waiting to be seen in the department they were attending. However nearly one in five patients said that the waiting area often got overcrowded, and there was some evidence to show that this was a particular problem in ophthalmic and dental clinics, in gynaecology, and in ear, nose and throat (ENT) clinics: an analysis showed that one in four patients attending these departments said they were often overcrowded.

As regards the seats themselves, again most patients (91%) found them satisfactory, although only half of this number were prepared to say they were actually comfortable. The main complaint was that the seats were too hard: it is this sort of seating, rather than low, soft, modern seating that is often preferred by elderly people, and it was therefore not surprising to find that younger patients were more likely to have found the seating in the waiting areas uncomfortable than older patients—see table 5.9 below.

Table 5.9 Proportion of patients in different age groups who found the seating in the waiting area uncomfortable

Patient found the seating	Patients aged:					
	0–16	17–34	35–54	55–64	65 and over	All ages
	%	%	%	%	%	%
comfortable	38	34	44	54	65	45
all right	51	54	47	41	32	46
uncomfortable	11	12	9	5	3	9
Base: all outpatients=100%[1]	511	468	511	302	374	2166

1. excludes patients in wheelchairs or on stretchers who could not comment

Indeed three of the 12 patients aged 65 or over who found the seats uncomfortable said this was because they were too soft.

54

Of all 186 patients who found the seats uncomfortable 39% specifically said this was because the seats were too hard, but we can probably add to this a further 24% who simply complained of wooden benches or wooden seats; indeed over half the reasons given as to why the seats were uncomfortable were concerned with their hardness. Five patients specifically complained that there was insufficient support for their backs, but again if the 24 patients who simply complained of sitting on benches, or backless chairs, are included 15% of patients were probably uncomfortable because of inadequate back support. Conversely however 13% of patients said the chairs were too upright. A similar proportion of patients (14%) said that the chairs were placed in rows too close together, giving insufficient leg room, and making it difficult for other patients to get past, and small proportions made comments such as there were no arms to the chairs, they were too high or simply that they were old fashioned. However it should be remembered that all these complaints came from less than 10% of the patients interviewed.

We then went on to ask what amenities were provided for patients and those accompanying them and as can be seen from the table below the level of provision was generally high.

Table 5.10 Provision of various amenities for outpatients and those accompanying them

Provision of amenity	Amenity			
	Refreshment facilities	Public telephone	Magazines/ newspapers to look at	Toys, games etc. for children[1]
	%	%	%	%
Provided	66	61	66	55
Not provided	21	9	23	45
Patient didn't know	13	30	11	—
Base: all outpatients= 100%[2]	2217	2218	2216	424

1. asked only of parents taking children under 14 as patients to hospital.
2. excludes 48 patients on stretchers who never used waiting rooms.

Just under half (46%) of the patients asked said there was a refreshment bar where people could get something to eat or drink (although in 5% of cases it was not usually open while they were at the hospital), 14% said there was a tea or coffee machine, and 5% that there was a trolley service. However in 11% of cases the patient said that other people might have difficulty in finding out where they could get a cup of tea. Similarly 5% of patients who knew there was a public telephone, either in the clinic they were attending or nearby, said that people might find it difficult to locate.

Although just under half the parents taking children to hospital said that nothing had been specially provided to keep children amused while they were waiting to be seen, almost all attending paediatric departments said that toys, games or comics were provided there for the children; parents taking children to casualty and outpatients were less likely to find these things available.

The demand for these amenities:

Although we were pleased to find that the amenities asked about had been available to many patients, the main concern was to find out what proportion of patients, who had not been able to get a cup of tea, or who had not had magazines to look at, would have found the time they had spent at hospital more pleasant had they been available. It was decided *not* to ask those who were not sure, or who did not know whether a particular facility was provided, whether they would have liked it to have been available; if for example, they really wanted a cup of tea, they would probably have found out whether or not it was possible to get one.

Apart from the provision of toys and games which nearly half the parents spoken to thought would have helped in keeping their children amused while they were waiting to be seen, there was only modest demand for the services asked about. The provision of magazines, books or newspapers in the waiting area received most support, from one in three of those attending departments where they were not available; one in four patients who had not been able to get anything to eat or drink would generally have liked to have been able to do so, and one in ten patients said it would have put their mind at rest had there been a public telephone either in the clinic they were attending or nearby.

As can be seen from the table below, the demand for these facilities consistently came from the younger patients. It may be of course that older people have different expectations as to what sort of facilities a hospital ought to provide for patients, or they may be more reluctant to appear dissatisfied than younger people, but nevertheless older patients and particularly those aged 65 or over, were far more likely than younger patients to say they were not bothered by the absence of these facilities.

Table 5.11 Proportions of patients in different age groups who would have liked various facilities to have been provided in or near the department they were attending

Patients aged	Facilities not available in dept. attended or nearby					
	Magazines in the waiting area		Refreshment facilities		A public telephone	
	%	Base= 100%	%	Base= 100%	%	Base= 100%
0–16	29	146	31	186	11	171
17–34	51	130	26	208	10	183
35–54	39	124	25	165	12	197
55–64	16	57	25	80	8	118
65 and over	7	61	15	107	7	142
All ages	33	518	25	746	10	811

1. Base: all for whom facility was not available in the dept. attended or nearby.

In the same way as the proportion of patients dissatisfied with the seating in the waiting area was, *overall,* very small, so it should also be remembered that partly because the facilities we asked about were generally available, the proportions "dissatisfied" because magazines, refreshments or a public telephone were not available represent comparatively small proportions of the total number of outpatients spoken to (7%, 8% and 4% respectively). Some patients were of course dissatisfied that, for example, there had been neither magazines to look at, nor somewhere to get a cup of tea, so by further analysis we found that overall 10% of people we spoke to were dissatisfied because at least one of these facilities had not been available.[19]

In chapter 7 we look in some detail at the length of time patients reported waiting before being seen by a doctor, and at their attitudes towards having to wait beyond their appointment time. We did however feel that the time the patient spent in the waiting area would almost certainly affect their views on comfort and on the facilities provided there. Analysis (see tables 5.12 and 5.13) confirmed that patients who had waited for comparatively long periods before being seen (about three quarters of an hour or longer) were more likely than those who spent shorter periods waiting to have found the seating uncomfortable, and to have wanted something to read, or eat and drink, or to have had access to a public telephone.

Table 5.12   **Proportions of patients waiting different lengths of time to be seen who would have liked certain facilities to have been provided in or near the department they were attending**

Time waited[1]	Facilities not available in dept. attended or nearby					
	Magazines in the waiting area		Refreshment facilities		A public telephone	
	%	Base= 100%[2]	%	Base= 100%[2]	%	Base= 100%[2]
up to 15 mins	24	257	17	441	8	486
about 30 mins	38	92	25	130	11	137
about 45 mins	43	42	39	54	11	57
about 1 hour or more	45	116	54	107	16	122

1. For patients who had a specific appointment time, the time waited is that beyond their actual appointment time.
2. Base=all for whom facility was not available in the dept. attended or nearby.

Table 5.13   **Proportions of patients waiting different lengths of time to be seen who found the seating in the waiting area uncomfortable**

Seating was:	Time waited to be seen[1]				
	5–10 mins	about 15 mins	about 30 mins	about 45 mins	about 1 hour or more
	%	%	%	%	%
comfortable	54	48	41	38	29
all right	41	46	49	51	54
uncomfortable	5	6	10	11	17
Base=100%[2]	879	363	380	168	343

1. for patients who had a specific appointment time, the time waited is that beyond their actual appointment time
2. base excludes patients on stretchers, or unconscious

19. Eight per cent of patients were dissatisfied that only one of the facilities asked about had not been available, 2% would have liked two out of the three facilities provided, and 0.2% would have liked to have been able to look at magazines, get a cup of tea and have a public telephone in or near the department they were attending.

For example it can be seen from table 5.13 above that while only 5% of patients who waited no more than about 15 minutes to be seen found the seats in the waiting area uncomfortable, this proportion rose to 17% among those who waited about an hour or more. Bearing in mind the length of wait involved it is perhaps surprising that this proportion is not even larger, and while we would wholeheartedly encourage the provision of comfortable seating, a more fundamental solution to the problem would be to make sure that patients do not have to sit for an hour or even longer before being seen.

Toilet facilities

The provision of toilets is a further facility that has not yet been discussed but which may be of more importance to patients than having magazines to look at, or being able to get a cup of tea, particularly for those patients who have had a long journey to hospital, or a long wait before being seen.

In asking about the toilet facilities at the hospital we were particularly interested in two aspects: their accessibility and their cleanliness.

Less than half (43%) the people spoken to had used the toilets at the hospital, but one in ten of those who had used them said they were difficult to find. Additionally there were nine patients who said they had not used the toilets because they were unable to find them, so that overall 6% of patients had difficulty in finding a toilet in or near the department they were attending. Generally however those who had used the toilets reported that they were clean (98%), that toilet paper was provided (only 2% remembered it not being available), and that there was somewhere to wash and dry their hands—95% remembered this being possible, 3% could not remember and 2% were sure it had not been possible.

Four patients who had not used the toilets said that was because they thought they might miss their turn, representing 0.2% of all the patients spoken to.

Having asked patients about the provision of certain specific facilities in the departments they were attending, they were then asked to comment overall on the appearance of the waiting area, and on its comfort.

About one in ten patients said they had not taken that much notice of its appearance, but of those who were able to comment, 15% found it *"a bit drab and depressing"* while the remainder were almost equally divided into those who had found it *"a bright and cheerful place to wait in"*, and those who were less enthusiastic but thought that *"it was all right"*.

Further analysis showed that paediatric departments were more likely than other departments to have been thought of as bright and cheerful, but that casualty and X-ray departments were thought of as drab and depressing more often than other departments.

The general comfort of the waiting areas in the departments was for most patients satisfactory: less than one in ten patients found it either very, or even rather, uncomfortable, and more than one in four had found it a very comfortable place to wait. However once again patients who had attended casualty were less enthusiastic about its comfort than those attending other departments or clinics—only 19% of patients attending casualty thought the waiting area was very comfortable.

Table 5.14   **Proportions of patients who were satisfied with the appearance of the waiting area in the department they had attended**

The waiting area was:	%	%
a bright and cheerful place	36	40
all right	41	45
a bit drab and depressing	14	15
patient didn't take much notice	9	
Base: all outpatients who used waiting room=100%	2213	2021[1]

1. excludes those who didn't take much notice of its appearance

Table 5.15   **Proportions of patients who found the waiting area in the department they had attended very comfortable**

Patients who found the waiting area:	%
very comfortable	28
all right	63
rather uncomfortable	7
very uncomfortable	2
Base: all outpatients who used the waiting area=100%	2214

The same patterns as were found previously when looking at patients' satisfaction with, and demand for, specific facilities, were found when looking more carefully at the patients who had an unfavourable view of the appearance of the waiting area, and at those who found it rather uncomfortable. Young people and those who waited for comparatively long periods before being seen were more likely to have had an unfavourable impression than older patients and those who only had a short time to wait before being seen. Women were also more likely to have noticed the appearance of the waiting area than men, and to have considered it more pleasant in appearance. These tables, together with tables which show that patients in higher social classes were more likely to have found the waiting areas drab and depressing and less likely to have found them comfortable, are to be found in Appendix III at the back of the report.

The further analyses, including those showing differences between patients from different social classes, may, as was suggested for the analyses that showed differences in the demand for certain facilities, reflect not only differences in patients' expectations, but also differences in their willingness to express dissatisfaction. Younger people and people from higher social classes may not only have different standards against which they compare the facilities for hospital patients, but it is likely that they are also more prepared than older people and those from lower social classes to voice their opinions and any dissatisfaction they feel.

5.3 Summary

The data presented in this chapter have shown that the majority of patients had access to the facilities and amenities that were asked about, and that where facilities were not provided, the demand for them came from less than half the patients spoken to. Widest support from inpatients came for the provision of a hospital shop or ward trolley service, and from outpatients for magazines or newspapers to be provided in waiting areas. Even here more than half of those who had not been able to buy sweets, cigarettes or toiletries while in hospital, and two out of three outpatients who had nothing to look at while waiting to be seen, were not bothered by the lack of these facilities.

The majority of outpatients were satisfied with the comfort and seating in the waiting area of the department they had attended, with its appearance and with the toilet facilities, although 6% of outpatients did say that other people might have difficulty in actually finding the toilets. Analysis showed that one in five outpatients found the waiting room both very comfortable and bright and cheerful in appearance, one in three said it was all right in appearance and comfort, and one in twenty found it drab and depressing and rather uncomfortable (see table 9 Appendix III).

A large proportion of the dissatisfaction that inpatients expressed with the washing and toilet facilities they had found while they were in hospital was the result of there being inadequate numbers of baths, showers and toilets for all who had to use them, and overall complaints about the washing and toilet facilities came from as many as one in five inpatients. Maternity patients were more likely to be dissatisfied with the bathing facilities: their needs are somewhat different from those of many other medical and surgical inpatients, and they were more likely to have found them inadequately catered for.

6.0 The hospital ward or room, its comfort and the daily routine
Inpatients only

This chapter is mainly concerned with two aspects of life in hospital: it describes the patients' daily routine—waking times, meals, and visiting sessions, shows how satisfied patients were with the various arrangements, and it looks at how comfortable the patient was in the physical surroundings of the room or ward they were in. We pay particular attention, later in the chapter, to the patients' views on the size of ward or room they were in, discussing the relative advantages and disadvantages of single rooms, small wards and large wards, and the chapter closes by showing what sort of ward a patient would prefer to be in, given the choice.

6.1 The daily routine in hospital

In talking to patients about various aspects of day-to-day life in hospital—meal times, waking times, visiting arrangements and so on, they were asked whether, when they were first admitted to hospital, the staff had explained the daily ward routine to them. We were somewhat surprised to find this did not seem to be a widespread practice: only 20% of all patients aged 14 and over said the daily routine had been explained to them. It was also interesting to find that men were more likely to have been told about the ward routine than women, and that maternity patients were the least likely group of patients to have been informed about day-to-day arrangements.

Table 6.1   Proportion of men and women patients who had the daily ward routine explained to them

Whether daily routine was explained to the patient:	Men	Women		Men and women
		maternity patients	non-maternity patients	
	%	%	%	%
Daily routine was explained	26	10	19	20
Daily routine was not explained	74	90	81	80
Base: all inpatients aged 14 and over=100%	242	97	358	697

However 40% of all patients (of all ages) said that before they were admitted to hospital they were sent a booklet or a leaflet which gave some information about the hospital, its facilities, arrangements for visiting and so on, and a further 19% said they were given such a booklet after they had been admitted. The data show that 35% of all adult patients had neither been given an explanatory booklet nor been told about the hospital routine by any of the staff. How important patients regarded being told about daily routine, and how useful they found the explanatory booklet is discussed in chapter 9 'Communication', but it seems that spending a few minutes with a patient soon after they have been admitted explaining the daily routine, would do a lot towards helping them settle down in hospital.

Perhaps two of the most popularly held beliefs about daily life in hospital are firstly that patients are woken extremely early in the morning, and secondly that the food in hospital is extremely poor. We looked to see if there was evidence to support these views.

Waking times

Table 6.2 below, confirmed that patients are generally woken quite early; over 40% of all patients were awake by 6.00 am. For maternity patients this proportion was even higher; 36% said they were awakened between 5.00 and 5.30 am, and 32% between 5.30 and 6.00 am.

Table 6.2 Times patients were generally woken in the morning

Patient was woken between . . .	Men	Women		Men and women
		maternity patients	non-maternity patients	
	%	%	%	%
5.00–5.30	7	36	8	12
5.31–6.00	34	32	30	32
6.01–6.30	32	19	37	32
6.31–7.00	20	6	17	16
7.01–7.30	7	5	6	6
7.31–8.00	*	2	1	1
after 8.00 am	—	—	1	1
Base: all inpatients aged 14 and over=100%	240	97	351	688

As many as a third of the patients awakened by 5.30 am felt that this was about the right time for them, but overall nearly half the patients complained of being woken too early (table 6.3).

Table 6.3 Proportions of patients woken at different times in the morning who felt they were woken too early

Patient was woken . . .	Patient was usually woken between					All
	5.00–5.30	5.31–6.00	6.01–6.30	6.31–7.00	after 7.00am	
	%	%	%	%	%	%
too early	67	47	46	27	17	43
too late	1	*	—	1	—	*
at about right time	32	53	54	72	83	57
Base: all inpatients aged 14 and over=100%	81	218	223	113	52	687

However, the proportion dissatisfied at being woken too early fell by nearly half among patients woken after 6.30 am; if therefore nursing staff could delay waking patients until after 6.30 am the proportion of patients complaining of being woken too early would be considerably reduced.

Further analysis showed that waking patients a bit later might be more appreciated on women's wards than on men's wards. Men, perhaps because they are more likely to have to get up early for work anyway, were less likely to complain of being woken too early than women: 35% of men said it was too early for them compared with 47% of women. There was no evidence that women with new babies who might have to be woken early for feeds felt differently to other women patients about the time they were woken in the morning.

Being woken very early in the morning may not matter quite so much if one has a good night's sleep or if it is possible to rest during the day.

Noise during daytime

More than one in ten (12%) of the adult patients spoken to, said they were disturbed by noise during the daytime, or found they were unable to rest if they wanted to do so (14%). As might have been expected, patients in smaller wards were less likely to have been disturbed by noise or been unable to rest than those in larger wards: about one in ten of those in wards with no more than ten beds said they were disturbed by noise, or were unable to rest during the daytime if they wished to do so, compared with nearly one in five of those in wards with more than 15 beds.

Further analysis also showed that women, and particularly maternity patients, were more likely to have been disturbed by noise, and to have found it difficult to rest than men patients. Many of the women who were in hospital to have a baby said that between feeding and changing their baby, being instructed in baby care, doing exercises and seeing visitors, they simply did not have time to rest during the day.

Overall of the 96 patients who would have liked to have been able to rest during the day, one in three said it was not possible because of the noise, and a similar proportion said that general activity in the ward such as meal times, visitors, and doctor's rounds, made it difficult to rest. One in four patients said they had not been allowed back to bed during the day and about one in ten said they were disturbed by cleaning staff, nurses and other hospital staff going about their work.

Disturbance during the night

While just over 10% of patients were unable to rest during the daytime if they wanted to do so, a much greater proportion (27%) said they were generally disturbed during the night, and for over half of these the disturbance was sufficient to make it difficult for them to get a fair night's sleep. Again, as can be seen from table 6.4 below, patients in the larger wards were more likely to have suffered than those in rooms or wards with only a small number of beds.

Table 6.4 Proportions of patients in hospital wards of different sizes who were disturbed at night and found it difficult to get a fair night's sleep

Disturbance at night	No. of beds in ward, or part of ward					All
	up to 4[1]	5–10	11–15	16–25	more than 25	
	%	%	%	%	%	%
Patient was not disturbed at night	80	76	71	63	64	73
Disturbance . . . made it difficult to sleep	9	11	25	24	26	16
was not that bad	11	13	4	13	10	11
Base: all inpatients aged 14 and over=100%	217	193	98	133	58	699

1. includes 38 patients who were in a room on their own throughout their stay in hospital

Less than one in ten of patients in small rooms with no more than four beds found it difficult to sleep, compared to one in four of those in wards for more than 15 patients. Once again men were less likely to be affected than women: one in five men said they were disturbed by noise and by things going on at night, compared to one in four women patients.

In many cases there is little that can be done about patients being disturbed during the night, especially for those in the larger wards; over half the patients spoken to who had difficulties said that the disturbance was caused by other patients in their ward, who snored, were in pain, or were otherwise restless, and about one in four said the disturbance was caused by patients being admitted as emergencies during the night. However, one in five patients disturbed by noise complained that the night staff made a noise, (banging doors and talking loudly) and a very small number of patients were disturbed by lights being kept on (either night lights in the ward, or on the nurse's table). A small number of patients mentioned being woken by nurses checking to see whether they were asleep (!), being disturbed by traffic noise outside the hospital, or being disturbed by machinery, including lifts and equipment outside their ward. One patient said the ward was infested by crickets.

Comfort of hospital beds

It may of course also be difficult to get a fair night's sleep if the bed is uncomfortable, and indeed, just under one in eight adults said that, bearing in mind their condition and the fact that it was a strange bed, they had found the hospital bed uncomfortable. The main cause of discomfort was the plastic drawsheet placed over the mattress. Nearly half of those who found their bed uncomfortable said this was the cause of the trouble; it was uncomfortable and it made them perspire.

Just over a third found their hospital bed too hard and about one in six said the height of the bed from the ground made it difficult to get in and out; maternity patients, both before delivery and after if they had had stitches, found this a particular problem. Among the other comments were several complaints from taller patients who said the hospital beds were too short for them and a number of comments about the sheets which were overstarched and consequently rough or stiff.

Table 6.5   Reasons why the hospital bed was found to be uncomfortable

Causes of discomfort	%
Rubber or plastic drawsheet	44
Bed was too hard	38
Bed was too high from the ground	17
Back rest uncomfortable when sitting	4
Complaints about pillows—too hard, not enough	3
Other reasons	37
Base: all who found their hospital bed uncomfortable=100%[1]	91

1. Percentages add to more than 100 as some people gave more than one reason

Temperature of ward

It has already been seen that a number of patients said they got uncomfortably hot in bed, and blamed this on the plastic drawsheet placed over the mattress; it was subsequently found that nearly a third of patients (30%) found that the ward or room they were in was generally kept too warm for them and indeed nearly half (45%) of the women in hospital to have a baby found it too warm. Overall only 6% of patients complained that generally their ward or room had not been kept sufficiently warm for them.

Meals and mealtimes in hospital

Three likely causes of complaints about hospital food were looked at; unsuitable mealtimes, lack of choice, and at the quality and serving of the food itself. In each of these areas a significant amount of dissatisfaction was found.

TIMES MEALS SERVED

Overall about one in four adult patients found that the meals were served at unsuitable times.

Maternity patients, whose mealtimes are doubtless affected by the feeding routines of their babies, were more likely than other women patients and men patients to have found the times that their own meals were served unsuitable in some way. Their complaints were also rather different to those of other patients. For example, many mothers said that their own meals were served while they were feeding their baby, and for one mother this had initially been a considerable problem. She had to go to the intensive care unit to feed her baby, and when she got back to the ward she found her meals had been left by her bed and were cold. However once she told the staff what was happening they put her meals in the oven for her to collect when she was ready. Maternity patients also complained that it seemed they had only just got to sleep themselves, after settling the baby from a 3.00 am feed, when they were woken for breakfast; indeed about 11% of patients woken before 6.00 am and 9% of all adult patients said breakfast was too early. About one in eight patients said they found it too long between their last meal at night and breakfast in the morning, some of whom said they had no

Table 6.6   Patients' opinions of the times that their meals were served while they were in hospital

Patients' opinions of times that meals were served	Men	Women maternity patients	non-maternity patients	Men and women
	%	%	%	%
Meals were served at suitable times:	74	65	76	74
Times were unsuitable . . . too long from last meal to breakfast	4	5	3	3
breakfast served too early	12	10	6	9
other meals served at awkward times	9	11	12	11
other answers	6	16	5	7
Base: all inpatients aged 14 and over=100%	239	96	356	691

supper or anything to drink after 6.30 p.m. A small number of patients complained that the first cup of tea came too early, largely reiterating their complaints at being woken too early, and a few felt that they waited too long between being woken and getting their breakfast.

TYPE OF MEAL

Apart from asking patients how they felt about the times that meals were served they were also asked whether they were generally satisfied or dissatisfied with the food. Although the popularly held impression is that hospital food is very poor, over three quarters of the adult patients spoken to said they were satisfied with the food and a similar proportion said there was a choice of dishes at mealtimes. If those patients who were on a diet are excluded, the proportion offered a choice of dishes rises to nearly 80%. A few patients did say however, that although they could choose from a menu, they were not always certain to get what they had ordered.

There is no evidence from this study that men were any more or less likely to have been dissatisfied with the food than women, nor that maternity patients held different opinions to other women patients. We thought that hospital food might perhaps be regarded as satisfactory if the stay in hospital is only a short one, and that as time passes one finds more shortcomings; however we found that patients in hospital for long periods (three weeks or more) were equally as satisfied as those who had been in for only a few nights.

Satisfaction with food

Overall the two main complaints about the food from those who were dissatisfied were that it was often cold by the time it reached them, and that it was tasteless or unattractive . . . *"it lacked colour and taste", "it was unappetising", ". . . food you could pick at but not eat with relish".* About one in four of those who were dissatisfied complained that the food was badly cooked in some way— lumpy potatoes, gravy and custard, and tough meat for example, and a similar proportion said the diet lacked variety. Men in particular, as can be seen from the table below, complained that the portions were too small, and indeed this was their chief cause of dissatisfaction. A small proportion of patients said that their particular needs—vegetarian meals, religious observations, were not adequately considered or catered for.

Table 6.7 Proportions of men and women who were dissatisfied with the food in hospital and the reasons for their dissatisfaction

Satisfaction with the food	Men		Women		Men and women	
	Nos	%	Nos	%	Nos	%
Satisfied with the food	260	85	392	80	652	82
Dissatisfied with the food	47	15	98	20	145	18
Base: all inpatients aged 14 and over=100%	307	100	490	100	797	100
Reasons for dissatisfaction:						
Base:[1] all dissatisfied with food	47	100%	98	100%	145	100%
food was served cold	11	23	41	42	52	36
no taste, unappetising	13	28	41	42	54	37
badly cooked	12	26	28	29	40	28
portions too small	16	34	17	17	33	23
not enough variety	10	21	25	26	35	24
specialist needs not considered	1	2	4	4	5	3
other reasons	14	30	30	31	44	30

1. Percentages add to more than 100 as some people gave more than one reason

A variety of other reasons for dissatisfaction were put forward, but each was mentioned by less than 1% of those dissatisfied: chief among these were complaints that the diet lacked fresh fruit and vegetables—*"everything was tinned, frozen or dehydrated"*, and complaints about the tea and coffee provided —it either tasted awful, or was not provided often enough, particularly after meals.

Visiting arrangements

DAYS AND TIMES
   Nearly all the adult patients (aged 14 and over) in the sample, said that while they were in hospital visitors had been allowed every day, including on Saturdays and Sundays; 3% said they had not been in hospital long enough to know about the visiting arrangements and 3% said visitors were permitted on only some days.[20] It can be seen from the table below that generally there were visiting sessions both in the afternoon and evening, indeed only 17 patients (2%) said there was no afternoon visiting at all, and by further analysis it was found that 388 patients (56%) were generally allowed visitors afternoons and evenings seven days a week.

Although visiting was generally allowed both in the afternoons and the evenings, on the occasions when it was not possible, most patients did not object. Over two thirds (69%) of those who could not have visitors in both the afternoon and the evening said that they personally would not have been in favour of it anyway.

20. Nine of the 18 patients who were not allowed visitors every day said visiting was allowed six days out of seven.

Not surprisingly most support for two visiting sessions a day came from maternity patients, while men were the least likely to be in favour of this suggestion.

Table 6.8   Proportions of patients generally being allowed visitors in the afternoons and in the evenings on the days when visiting was allowed

On visiting days visitors were allowed	On visiting days visitors were allowed:			All patients 14 and over
	every evening	only on some evenings	no evening sessions	
	%	%	%	%
Every afternoon	60	1	—	61
Only on some afternoons	29	8	—	37
No afternoon sessions	2	—	—	2
All	91	9	—	100[1]

1. Base: all inpatients aged 14 and over who knew when visiting sessions were=667=100%

Table 6.9   Proportions of men and women who would have liked visiting sessions in the afternoon and in the evening on the days when visitors were allowed

Whether would have liked afternoon and evening visiting	Men	Women		Men and women
		maternity patients	non-maternity patients	
	%	Nos.	%	%
Yes, would have liked two sessions	23	[15]	34	31
No, would not have liked this	77	[19]	66	69
Base:[1]=100%	102	34	149	285

1. Base: all inpatients aged 14 and over who were not allowed visitors in both the afternoon and evening on visiting days.

Nine out of ten patients said that on the whole the visiting hours were convenient for their own visitors (the chief complaint being that visiting hours were not always completely outside working hours), but one in eight would have liked the sessons to have been longer. Thirty eight patients (5%) would have preferred shorter visiting hours. Although the numbers were small, again there was some evidence that maternity patients were in favour of longer visiting sessions, while men were more likely to have preferred shorter hours.

NUMBER OF VISITORS

Just under half (46%) of the patients said that in practice generally no limit was put on the number of visitors they were allowed to have;[21] nearly all the other patients were generally restricted to two visitors at a time. Where there was a restriction, most patients felt that it was set at about the right number, but there was a difference of opinion as to whether there should always be a restriction on

21. We found that a somewhat greater proportion of patients who had been in hospital for three weeks or more said that there was no limit on the number of visitors they were allowed, compared to those in hospital for shorter periods. This suggests that rules are perhaps relaxed for patients who are in hospital for comparatively long periods.

the number of visitors allowed. Overall there was more support for there being no restriction on the numbers of visitors allowed (61% of patients held this view) but patients in wards where there *had* been a limit on numbers were more in favour of restrictions than those who had no restrictions on the number of visitors while they were in hospital. Two thirds of patients whose own visitors had been limited were in favour of such restrictions compared with just over a third of those whose visitors had not been limited in number. There appeared to be no association between the age or sex of the patient or the size of the ward they had been in, and their views on whether the number of visitors should be limited.

VISITS BY CHILDREN

Nearly three quarters (72%) of inpatients said that children were allowed to visit in the ward they were in, although in just under half of these cases it was restricted to certain visiting sessions. On balance, patients were generally in favour of children being allowed to visit in hospital, although nearly two thirds of the 572 patients supporting the suggestion did have reservations. Overall 13% were totally against the idea of children being allowed to visit and 5% did not particularly mind one way or the other; 31% were in favour of children being allowed to visit at any session and the remaining 51% were in favour but on certain conditions. Further analysis showed that women in hospital to have babies were the most likely to give their unconditional support to children visiting, and perhaps surprisingly, as many men were in favour of the idea as women. However, as can be seen from the table below, older patients, and particularly those aged 65 and over, were more likely to be against children being allowed to visit; one in five patients aged 65 and over were totally against the idea, compared with less than one in ten of patients aged under 35.

Table 6.10: Proportions of patients in different age groups in favour of children being allowed to visit in hospital

Attitude to children being allowed to visit in hospital	Patients aged				
	14–34	35–54	55–64	65 & over	All ages
	%	%	%	%	%
In favour—no reservations	36	27	32	26	31
In favour—only with reservations	50	60	45	45	51
Against	9	11	16	20	13
Not bothered	5	2	7	9	5
Base: all inpatients aged 14 and over=100%	261	195	102	138	696

About half of the patients who were against children being allowed to visit, said this was because they felt it was too upsetting for children to see people who were ill. Just under a third said that generally children could not be controlled adequately and would be disturbing, and about one in five thought that the children could either bring infections into the ward or catch infections while they were there. As can be seen from the table below, those who had reservations about children visiting had much the same considerations in mind; children should only be allowed as visitors *if* they could be kept under control, *if* they were not upset by it, *if* they were healthy themselves and so on.

Table 6.11: Conditions under which children should be allowed to visit

Conditions under which children should be allowed to visit	%
if they are kept under control	46
if the patient being visited is well enough	35
only "older" children allowed	19
if the child is not upset by seeing ill people	17
only patients' own children allowed	11
the child must be healthy—no colds	4
other answers	6
Base: all in favour of children being allowed to visit in hospital, but with reservations=100%[1]	356

1. Percentages add to more than 100 as some people gave more than one condition.

Patients' attitudes to smoking in hospital

Although nearly half the adult patients spoken to said that patients were not allowed to smoke in the room or hospital ward they were in and had to go elsewhere in the hospital if they wanted to smoke, nevertheless as many as one in three patients said that smoking was permitted in their ward. As might have been expected maternity patients were the least likely to have been allowed to smoke in their own room or ward, but as can be seen from the table below even non-maternity women patients were less likely than men patients to have been permitted to smoke in their room or hospital ward.

Table 6.12: Proportions of men and women who were allowed to smoke in the hospital ward or room they were in.

Restrictions on patients smoking in hospital	Men	Women		Men and women
		maternity patients	non-maternity patients	
	%	%	%	%
Could smoke in ward	44	24	30	34
Had to go elsewhere to smoke	41	68	49	49
Not allowed to smoke in hospital at all	6	1	4	4
Did not know whether smoking was allowed	9	7	17	13
Base: all inpatients aged 14 and over =100%	242	97	360	699

We were particularly interested to find out how patients felt about being allowed, or not being allowed to smoke in their ward and in seeing whether there was any one group that felt strongly about this issue.

Overall a comparatively small minority of patients (14%) were either unhappy at not being allowed to smoke, or pleased that they had been allowed to smoke in their ward (we call this group those *in favour of smoking*). The remaining patients were then equally divided into those who were either pleased that patients had not been permitted to smoke, or objected to smoking having been allowed (those *in favour of no smoking*) and a group that did not mind one way or the other. As the table below shows, women in general, and particularly maternity patients and younger patients were more likely to be in favour of a ban on smoking than either men or older patients.

Table 6.13: Patients' attitudes towards being allowed to smoke in their own room or hospital ward.

Attitude to smoking in the hospital ward	Men	Women		Men and women aged:				Men and women		All men and women
		maternity patients	non-maternity patients	14–34	35–54	55–64	65 and over	smokers	non-smokers	
	%	%	%	%	%	%	%	%	%	%
In favour of *no smoking*	28	65	47	51	38	47	33	30	55	43
In favour of *smoking*	19	4	13	12	17	10	14	27	2	14
Didn't mind either way	53	31	40	37	45	43	53	43	43	43
Base: all patients aged 14 and over=100%	217	96	291	228	178	91	107	281	323	604

Naturally enough patients who were themselves smokers were more likely to be in favour of being allowed to smoke in the ward than non-smokers, only 2% of whom were in favour of smoking being allowed in the ward. Among smokers support came from one in four overall and from one in three of the men patients who smoked; over half the men patients who were smokers said that they did not mind either way whether or not they were allowed to smoke in their ward.

6.2 Patients' views on the size of the ward they were in

The wards and rooms that patients were in during their spell in hospital have already been described and it has been seen that just over half the adult patients spent at least some of their time in fairly small wards with no more than ten beds, and that less than 10% had been in large wards for more than 25 patients.[22] Nine out of ten patients (excluding those who had spent their entire time in a single room on their own) said they thought there were about the right number of beds in the ward or part of the ward they were in, but as would probably be expected there were more who thought there were too many beds—66 patients—than who thought there were too few—six patients. Dissatisfaction, not surprisingly, was directly related to the number of beds in the ward; less than one in twenty of patients in wards with no more than ten beds felt this was too many compared with one in three of those in wards with more than 25 beds. Given that men were more likely to have been in a large ward than women, it was interesting to find that there were no significant differences between men and women in the proportions thinking their wards too large.

Table 6.14   Proportions of men and women in wards of different sizes who thought their ward had too many beds

No. of beds in ward was:	No. of beds in ward/part of ward					Men	Women	All
	up to 4	5–10	11–15	16–25	over 25			
	%	%	%	%	%	%	%	%
too many	2	3	9	20	35	11	9	10
too few	2	1	2	—	—	1	1	1
about right	96	96	89	80	65	88	90	89
Base=100%[1]	178	193	98	132	57	233	425	658

Base: all inpatients aged 14 and over=100%

It would seem from the information collected that a 15-bedded ward is the maximum size that most patients will be happy in, larger than this, (and over a quarter of all adult patients had been in wards with more than 15 beds) and the proportion of dissatisfied patients increases considerably.

A third of those who thought their ward was too large felt there were too many patients for the nursing staff to cope with; these two comments were typical:

"It was too many for the nursing staff. They had too much to do, nobody was neglected but the nurses were overworked".

". . . too much to cope with, in the nights (there was) always someone shouting out and not enough nurses to cope with it".

22. see p.47—chapter 5.

Half the patients said they felt squashed or overcrowded with not enough room between the beds, which might suggest that there were more beds in the ward than it was originally designed to take, and a small but significant number of patients (13 of the 66) said the noise was too much for them, particularly when they did not feel very well, or they found there was constant disturbance. Additionally small numbers of patients mentioned a lack of privacy, or inadequate washing and toilet facilities for the number of patients that needed to use them (both of these are topics discussed elsewhere). Finally two people had been distressed by seeing seriously ill and dying patients on their ward: they felt this was less likely to happen on a smaller ward.

Two of the six patients who felt there were too few beds on their ward would have liked more company, and three (with no mention of other considerations) felt that as there were always people waiting for admission to hospital there should be more beds in the wards. However one patient in saying why she felt there were too few beds in her ward presented another aspect of the problem nursing staff face in coping with large numbers of patients no matter how hospital wards or rooms are designed. . . .

"Because the available beds were split into small groups the nursing staff were not able to keep sight of patients to any degree of reassurance".

Patients' preferences

All patients aged 14 and over were asked the following question . . . *"Thinking back to your own experience as a patient, if you had to go into hospital again, would you prefer to be in a room on your own, in a small ward with up to about six beds, or in a ward with more than about six beds?".* They were then asked the reason for their choice. Given the alternatives, it was not surprising to find that nearly two thirds opted for *'a small ward with up to about six beds',* see table 6.15 below.

Table 6.15   Type of hospital ward preferred by men and women in different age groups

Patients' preference	Age groups				Men	Women	All
	14–34	35–54	55–64	65 and over			
	%	%	%	%	%	%	%
a room on their own	7	14	11	13	10	11	11
a small ward with up to about 6 beds	71	60	62	49	58	64	62
a ward with more than about 6 beds	22	26	27	38	32	25	27
Base: all inpatients aged 14 and over =100%[1]	258	190	103	130	233	448	681

1. excludes the 18 patients who could not choose or were not bothered.

One quarter preferred the larger ward (although we suspect from previous information that few would choose to be in a ward with more than about 15 beds), and one in ten given the choice would opt for a room of their own. Eight people definitely would not want to be on their own but could not choose between the other two alternatives, and ten patients said they were not bothered at all. There were no differences between the choices made by men and by women, although women who had been in hospital to have a baby were rather more likely to prefer to be in a small ward with up to about six beds than other women patients: the proportions were 79% and 59% respectively.[23] As can be seen from the table above there were however differences in the preferred options of patients in different age groups.

Small wards were the favourite choice for patients in every age group, but particularly among the younger patients, nearly three quarters of whom would prefer to be in a small ward with up to six beds. However this preference was not nearly so marked among the elderly; less than half the patients aged 65 and over preferred the small ward, but well over a third (38%) said they would choose to be in a larger ward with more than six beds, a much greater proportion than among any other age group.

Because only a limited number of options were actually put to patients it was difficult to see how far patients' expressed preferences coincided with their actual experiences. It can however be seen from the table below that half of those in a room on their own would have made that choice anyway, and that 82% of those in the smallest wards—not more than four beds—would opt for the same again.

Reasons for preferring a particular size of ward, or a single room

It has already been seen that a number of patients found it difficult to rest during the day and difficult to get a fair night's sleep because of noise, it was not surprising therefore to find that over half (52%) of the 74 patients who, given the choice, would opt for a room on their own said this was because it would be quieter. Preferring not to see other ill people or hear about their complaints or operations was mentioned by 18%, and one in four admitted to simply preferring their own company or not being particularly sociable. More privacy was a deciding factor for a considerable proportion of patients (20%) either when being examined or treated or when visitors were there, and a small number of informants thought there was more freedom for patients in single rooms— visiting arrangements would be more flexible, they could choose which TV programme to watch, and so on.

Almost all the 184 patients who preferred to be in a ward with more than about six beds gave the same reason in support of their choice: 180 opted for the larger ward because they felt it was better to have company and to always have things going on around them to stop them getting bored or depressed and, in particular, they preferred to have a wider choice of patients to talk to and make friends with than would be possible in a smaller ward. In addition there were a number of other interesting reasons put forward but each was only mentioned by very few patients. Seven patients, expressing a view contrary to that found earlier, said they felt they would get better attention in a larger ward. . . .

". . . there's more chance of catching the nurses if you need something because they're in and out of larger wards rather than small ones".

---

23. Even when we compared women of similar ages, those who had gone into hospital to have a baby were still more likely to have preferred a small ward with up to six beds than other women patients.

Table 6.16 Size of ward that patient was in on this occasion compared with the type of ward they would prefer to be in on any future occasion

Type of ward patient would prefer in future	Size of ward patient was in on this occasion												All inpatients aged 14 and over	
	Single room on own		Number of beds											
			up to 4		5–10		11–15		16–25		more than 25			
	Nos	%	Nos	%	Nos	%	Nos	%	Nos	%	Nos	%	Nos	%
a room on their own	20	3	19	3	16	2	6	1	8	1	5	1	74	11
small ward with up to 6 beds	13	2	141	21	141	21	51	7	52	8	25	4	423	62
ward with more than 6 beds	4	*	16	2	32	5	40	6	67	10	25	4	184	27
All inpatients aged 14 and over	37	5	176	26	189	28	97	14	127	19	55	8	Base: 681=100%	

75

Three patients felt they would be reassured by knowing that there were always other patients around to summon help in an emergency, and a similar number mentioned the assistance and reassurance that patients can give each other, including by being able to see other patients with more serious or similar conditions to their own making good recoveries.

Being in a small ward with up to about six beds, is, of course, the compromise between the isolation of being in a room on one's own, and the activity of a large ward, and naturally the reasons patients gave for preferring the smaller ward reflected this. As can be seen from the table below, of all the patients making this choice over 80% mentioned that it would be better and preferable for them not to be on their own but to have company, about half this number said a small ward would be less noisy than a larger ward and about one in ten said they would have more privacy. On looking more closely at this group of patients (table 6.17 below) differences were found in the frequency with which these reasons were given by men and by women and by older patients compared to young people.

Table 6.17   Reasons for preferring to be in a small ward with up to about six beds rather than in a larger ward or a single room: men and women in different age groups.

Reasons for preferring to be in a small ward	Age groups				All men	All women	Men and women
	14–34	35–54	55–64	65 and over			
	%	%	%	%	%	%	%
Better to have company	88	88	83	75	84	86	85
Less noise	35	53	39	28	47	36	39
More privacy	14	11	8	5	7	13	11
More attention from nursing staff	11	8	8	5	11	8	9
Not with seriously ill patients	2	5	5	6	3	4	4
Other reasons	8	5	8	20	8	9	9
Base: all preferring to be in a small ward=100%[1]	181	112	64	64	135	286	421

1. Percentages add to more than 100 as some people gave more than one reason.

A much greater proportion of men, compared with woman, were concerned that the ward should be quiet (47% and 36% respectively). Women and younger patients were however more likely to mention the better privacy that a smaller ward could offer than men and patients aged 55 and over. It has already been seen that there were a few patients who felt they would get better attention from nursing staff in a larger ward, here we found 9% of patients who felt the same way, but about smaller wards. . . .

"You get better treatment—in a large ward it takes them all their time to get round when they bring you the medicines".

"If there's a lot of beds you can't get the same attention, it stands to sense the nurses have more to see to".

While a few of those preferring larger wards found it reassuring to see others with more serious illnesses than their own recovering, 4% of this group definitely did not want to be with patients who were seriously ill, and thought there was less chance of this happening in a smaller ward. . . .

"A big ward with a lot of people in pain is off-putting"

"In a big ward you often see more serious illness. I found it frightening".

7.0 Outpatient appointments and waiting to see the doctor
Outpatient sample only

It has already been shown that patients who spent comparatively long periods waiting at the hospital before being seen were less likely than patients who waited only a short time before being seen to have had a favourable impression of the waiting area, and more likely to have wanted certain amenities provided for them and those accompanying them to hospital. This chapter looks in more detail at how long patients spent waiting to be seen by a doctor at the hospital: in particular the patients' own opinions of the appointment system and how well the system appeared to be working are examined. How long patients expect to have to wait to be seen, what leads them to hold these opinions, and how far their expectations were borne out by their own experience are also discussed.

7.1 Patients with appointments

Of course not all patients had attended hospital by appointment; 436 of the 2267 patients who were interviewed said that the only visit—or indeed all the visits—they had made to hospital in connection with the condition under discussion had been made without an appointment. It was not possible therefore to ask them whether or not they found their appointments convenient. However of the 1831 patients who had attended by appointment, only 5% found their appointments inconvenient, 45% had been given some say in fixing the appointment anyway, and the remainder (50%) although having no say themselves, said the times they were given were usually satisfactory. Although 1831 patients had attended hospital by appointment, not all were given specific appointment times: 179 patients were told that they could, for example, go along at any time on a particular day or attend any day between certain times: these are subsequently referred to as patients with *open appointments*. These 179 patients with open appointments were no less likely than those with specific appointment times to have been given a say in fixing their appointment nor were they any more likely to have found them satisfactory (table 7.1).

Table 7.1 **Proportions of patients with specific appointment times who had a say in fixing their appointments and who usually found them satisfactory.**

Patients' satisfaction with appointment times	Appointments were		All attending by appointment
	for specific times	open	
	%	%	%
Patient had a say in fixing appointment	45	46	45
Patient had no say . . .			
but appointment given was usually satisfactory	49	50	50
and would have preferred different appointment	6	4	5
Base: all attending by appointment=100%	1652	179	1831

Patients said that the inconvenience was generally caused by the appointment either being during working hours, or being at a time when children had to be taken or collected from school. It was therefore not surprising to find that men and women with jobs, and mothers with children aged under 11 were the two groups most likely to have said that they would have preferred their appointments to have been fixed for different times (see tables 10 and 11 Appendix III).

Arriving early for an appointment

Just over half the 1652 patients with specific appointments said they usually managed to arrive within 5 or 10 minutes of their appointment time, but two out of every five said they usually got there earlier than that. A very small proportion said they were more than about 10 minutes late and it was interesting to find (table 7.2 below) that these were more likely to have been patients who were always taken to hospital by ambulance or hospital car than patients who made their own way there.

Table 7.2   Proportions of patients who made their own way to hospital or were taken by ambulance who usually arrived within about 5 or 10 minutes of their appointment time

Patient usually arrived at hospital . . .	How patient got to the hospital			All
	always used hospital transport	sometimes used hospital transport	always made own way	
	%	%	%	%
within 5 or 10 mins of appointment	49	43	59	57
was earlier than that	37	51	40	41
was usually late	14	6	1	2
Base: all outpatients given specific appointment times=100%	126	91	1426	1643

Nearly half of those arriving more than about 10 minutes before their appointment time said they liked to leave themselves plenty of time so as not to risk being late, but arriving early was not always a matter of choice: one in four said they had no option as the transport got there early and closer inspection showed that many of these were patients who arrived by ambulance. Even if ambulance patients are excluded then 16% of patients making their own way to hospital for specific appointments had no option, because of the transport, other than to arrive early.

As can be seen from table 7.3 one in five patients arriving early said this was because they thought they might be seen before their appointment time, but it was perhaps more interesting to find that a slightly greater proportion, 22%, got to hospital early because they thought they would be *'first in the queue'*, implying that they believed several patients were given the same appointment time as themselves and that by arriving early they might be the first to be seen of all those booked for that particular time. When asked directly, 48% of all patients given a specific appointment said they thought that other patients were also being asked to come along at the same time as they had been given. Only 36% of patients thought they had a personal and individual appointment time, and the remaining 16% said they had never given the issue any thought.

Table 7.3   Reasons why patients with specific appointment times usually arrived more than about 10 minutes early for their appointment

Reasons why patients arrived early for their appointments	%
Like to leave plenty of time	48
Transport arrives early—no option	23
Thought might be seen before appointment time	19
Thought would be first in the queue	22
Other reasons	4[1]
Base: all outpatients arriving early for specific appointments=100%[2]	669

1. includes three patients who said the hospital asked patients to arrive about 15 minutes before their appointment.
2. proportions add to more than 100 as some patients gave more than one reason.

As can be seen from table 7.4 analysis confirmed that patients who thought they were given the same appointment time as other patients were more likely to get to the hospital early than patients who thought their appointment time was particular to them alone.

Table 7.4   Proportions of patients who arrived early for their appointment

Patient usually arrived at hospital	Patient thought that they were given		All with specific appointment times
	an individual appointment time	the same appointment time as other patients	
	%	%	%
within 5 or 10 mins of appointment	61	53	57
was earlier than that	37	44	41
was usually late	2	3	2
Base: all outpatients with specific appointment times=100%	594	780	1637[1]

1. the 263 patients who had never considered whether other patients might have been given the same appointment time as their own are included in this column.

7.2   How long did patients expect to have to wait before being seen?

Patients with appointments fixed for specific times were asked how long after their appointment time they expected to have to wait before being seen. Those who had open appointments, or no appointment at all were asked how long they thought they might have to wait to be seen from the time they arrived at the hospital. A number of patients, particularly those attending as casualties or without an appointment were unable to answer this question as they had been unconscious or otherwise unaware of their situation at the time. However, as can

Table 7.5 How long patients expected to have to wait before being seen

Patient expected to wait . . .	Patients with appointments				Patients with no appointments	
	for specific times		open appointments			
	Nos	%	Nos	%	Nos	%
about 5 or 10 minutes	536	36	49	34	88	27
about 15 minutes	238	16	29	20	41	12
about 30 minutes	333	23	31	21	81	25
about 45 minutes	82	5	9	6	15	5
between about 1 and 2 hours	163	11	27	18	100	30
more than about 2 hours	—	—	1	1	3	1
thought would be seen before appointment time	126	9	—	—	—	—
Base: all outpatients=100%	1478[1]	100	146[2]	100	328[3]	100

1. excludes 140 patients who thought they would have to wait more than about 5 or 10 minutes, but had no idea of how much longer.
2. excludes 30 patients who were either unconscious or had no idea of how long they would have to wait.
3. excludes 80 patients who were either unconscious or had no idea of how long they would have to wait.

be seen from table 7.5, overall about one in three patients expected to be seen quickly—within 5 or 10 minutes of their appointment time or of arriving at the hospital.

Generally however, as might be expected, patients with appointments for specific times expected to be seen more quickly than either patients with open appointments or than those with no appointments at all. The table shows that nearly one in three patients attending without an appointment expected a wait of between one and two hours, and these 100 patients represent 4% of all outpatients spoken to in the course of this study.

There was no evidence to suggest that older patients were less likely than younger patients to expect to be seen quickly, but it was very clear that previous experience played a considerable part. As can be seen from table 7.6, two thirds of those who expected to have to wait at least an hour said that their own previous personal experience, either as a patient or when accompanying someone else to hospital, led them to believe that they would have to wait that long.

Table 7.6   Reasons why patients expected to have to wait more than 5 or 10 minutes after their appointment time or after arriving at the hospital before being seen

Reasons why patients expected to have to wait:	Patient expected to wait:				All
	about 15 mins	about 30 mins	about 45 mins	about 1 hour or longer	
	%	%	%	%	%
own previous experience	43	46	55	67	51
experience of friends/ relatives	2	4	3	4	3
'common knowledge'	19	16	15	11	15
many patients already waiting	26	12	30	24	21
time between appointments too short	16	14	5	3	11
expect serious cases to be seen first	11	10	7	8	9
several patients given same appointment time	4	6	7	4	5
hospital are short of staff	3	3	7	5	4
doctors not always available	4	4	3	5	4
other answers	9	4	3	7	6
Base: all outpatients who expected to wait more than 5 or 10 mins to be seen=100%[1]	294	441	106	290	1131

1. percentages add to more than 100 as some patients gave more than one reason.

Overall over half the patients based their expectations on their own personal experience or that of friends or relatives, and the majority of the patients gave no other reasons to support their view. Many other reasons were given however, and indeed the appointment system itself was often blamed for causing delays.

This can be seen more clearly from table 7.7 which shows the reasons why patients with specific appointment times expected to have to wait to be seen, and the reasons given by those who had open appointments or no appointments at all.

Table 7.7 Reasons why patients expected to have to wait more than 5 or 10 minutes after their appointment time, or after arriving at the hospital before being seen: those with specific appointments and those with open, or no appointments at all

Reasons why patients expected to have to wait	Those with specific appointment times	Those with open appointments or no appointments at all
	%	%
own previous experience	55	44
experience of friends/relatives	3	5
'common knowledge'	10	28
time between appointments too short	15	NA[1]
several patients given same appointment time	7	NA[1]
appointments made when doctors not available	4	NA[1]
many patients already waiting	23	35
expect serious cases to be seen first	8	12
hospitals are short of staff	4	5
doctors not always available	—	4
other answers	6	5
Base: all outpatients who expected to wait more than 5 or 10 mins to be seen=100%[2]	801	330

1. NA=not applicable
2. percentages add to more than 100 as some patients gave more than one reason

About one in seven patients with specific appointments said that the time allowed between one appointment and the next was too short, leading to delays, and about half this number thought the delays were due to several patients being booked for the same appointment time.[24] A few patients also felt the hospital was at fault in making appointments for patients when doctors would generally not be available—early morning appointments and appointments during the lunch hour were given as examples.

Many patients naturally enough estimated how long they would have to wait from the number of other patients already waiting to be seen; about one in four of those with specific appointments and one in three of those with open appointments or no appointments at all said many patients were already there when they arrived, whom, they assumed, would have to be seen before their own turn came.

Tables 12 and 13 in Appendix III give, in full, the reasons patients gave for expecting to have to wait to be seen, analysed by type of appointment and length of expected wait.

24. It has already been seen that about half the patients with specific appointments thought they had been told to attend at the same time as other patients.

7.3　How long patients actually waited before being seen

The data showed that over 40% of outpatients reported that on their last visit to hospital, they had been seen within about 5 or 10 minutes either way of their appointment time, or of arriving at the hospital, and that three quarters had been seen within about 30 minutes (table 7.8).

Table 7.8　How long patients, on their last visit to hospital, had actually waited before being seen

| Patient actually waited . . . | Patients with appointments | | | | Patients with no appointments | | All | |
| | for specific times | | open appoint- ments | | | | | |
	%	cum%	%	cum %	%	cum %	%	cum %
no more than about 5 or 10 mins	42	42	40	40	42	42	42	42
about 15 mins	16	58	18	58	19	61	17	59
about 30 mins	18	76	20	78	14	75	18	77
about 45 mins	8	84	7	85	8	83	8	85
between about 1 and 2 hours	14	98	15	100	17	100	14	99
more than about 2 hours	2	100	—		—		1	100
Base: all outpatients =100%[1]	1627		175		424		2226	

1. excludes those unconscious or dazed

However, as can be seen from the table, some 15% of all outpatients waited more than about an hour to be seen, and 2% of those with specific appointment times reported waiting more than about two hours before being attended to.

It was particularly interesting to find that patients with open appointments, and those with no appointments at all had generally waited no longer to be seen than patients who had been given specific appointment times.

By looking at how long patients generally expected to have to wait and at their actual experiences (tables 7.5 and 7.8) it can be seen that patients with no appointments at all tended to overestimate considerably how long they would have to wait: only about a quarter thought they would be seen within 5 or 10 minutes whereas over 40% were actually seen that quickly. For patients with open appointments the distribution of answers as to how long they expected to have to wait resembles quite closely what actually happened, while for patients with specific appointments there appeared to be some tendency to underestimate the waiting time. More detailed analysis which compared each patient's estimate with how long they actually waited showed that 46% of patients with specific appointments were accurate in their estimate of how long they would wait, as were 43% of those with open appointments, and only 28% of those with no appointment at all. As can be seen from table 7.9 below this more detailed analysis confirmed that of all those who were incorrect in their estimates, patients with specific appointment times were more likely to underestimate how long they would have to wait than either of the other two groups.

Table 7.9 Proportions of patients who overestimated how long they would have to wait to be seen

Comparison of patient's estimate and actual wait on last visit to hospital	Patients with appointments		Patients with no appointments
	for specific times	open appointments	
	%	%	%
patient overestimated length of wait	47	58	64
patient underestimated length of wait	53	42	36
Base=100%[1]	791	83	231

1. Base=all outpatients who were incorrect in their estimate of how long they would have to wait to be seen.

Patients who thought they waited an unreasonable length of time to be seen

Less than 5% of patients who, on their last visit to hospital, waited about 15 minutes or longer to be seen, said that when they arrived at the hospital they had been told how long they might have to wait to be seen and only one in ten said they were given an explanation as to why they had to wait.

The original data show that 28% of those who waited more than about 15 minutes felt this was an unreasonable length of time to have to wait, but further analysis (table 7.10 below) showed that patients with specific appointments were more likely than patients who had open appointments to regard waiting 15 minutes or longer before being seen as unreasonable.

Table 7.10 Proportions of patients with specific appointments, open appointments, and no appointments at all who regarded a wait of 15 minutes or more as unreasonable

Waiting 15 minutes or longer to be seen was . .	Patients with appointments		Patients with no appoint-ments	All waiting 15 minutes or longer
	for specific times	open appointments		
	%	%	%	%
reasonable	70	83	73	72
unreasonable	30	17	27	28
Base=100%[1]	938	103	244	1285

1. Base=all outpatients who waited 15 minutes or longer before being seen

Indeed patients who had open appointments, were the least likely to be dissatisfied at having to wait to be seen, despite the fact that, as has already been shown, they waited as long before being seen as other patients.

It was not surprising to find that the proportion of dissatisfied patients increased in direct proportion to the length of wait. As can be seen from table 7.11 below, there was a substantial increase in the porportion regarding the wait as unreasonable, between those who waited about 15 minutes and those who waited about 30 minutes, and again for those who waited an hour or longer.

Table 7.11 Proportions of patients who waited about 15 minutes or longer to be seen on their last visit to hospital who felt the wait was unreasonable

Patients' opinion of length of wait	Length of time patient waited before being seen				All waiting 15 mins or longer
	about 15 mins	about 30 mins	about 45 mins	about 1 hr or longer	
	%	%	%	%	%
wait was unreasonable	6	38	35	60	28
wait was not unreasonable	94	62	65	40	72
Base=all who waited 15 mins or longer=100%	371	386	172	348	1277

There was some evidence that patients who had been told how long they might have to wait were less likely to find the wait unreasonable than those who had not been told what to expect: the proportions were 15% and 29% respectively.[25] Moreover, nearly half (46%) of those who had not been told how long a wait to expect said that being told might have helped; in fact only a comparatively small proportion of these patients (16%) actually asked.

When patients were asked why they had not enquired as to how long they could expect to wait before being seen, over a third said they had not bothered because they felt there would be no point, they just had to wait their turn. A further 24% said that they simply *"had not thought of doing so"*, but 6% had wanted to do so but said they could not find anyone to ask. A small, but nevertheless significant, proportion of patients had decided not to ask how long they could expect to wait for various reasons connected with what they saw as the attitude of the staff: 6% had not asked because they felt the staff were too busy to be bothered, 4% said they were put off by the attitude of the staff, for example one patient said. . . .

"the nurse was not particularly pleasant, you thought she might snap back at you",

and another . . .

"the receptionist wasn't very nice, she was doing you a favour just to speak to you",

and finally a very small number of patients (1% of those not asking) said they had not asked how long they might have to wait before being seen because they thought to do so might adversely affect their relationship with the staff . . .

"well it might put their backs up. I wouldn't want them to be unkind or brusque to the child thinking I was unpleasant."

"I didn't want to be unpleasant because it might affect your treatment: the doctor might be unkind to you when you see him."

The relationship between doctors, other hospital staff and patients and, in particular, the willingness of patients to ask questions and to get answers which are to their satisfaction, is examined in more detail in a later chapter.

---

25. There was no relationship between being told how long the wait might be and the actual length of time waited.

7.4 Type of appointment preferred by outpatients

Three out of every four outpatients interviewed said that if they were given a choice, they would prefer a specific appointment time; one in eight would prefer to be told to go along at any time between certain hours—an open appointment—and the remaining one in ten said they had no preference.

Although, as has already been shown, on their last visit to hospital many outpatients with specific appointments felt they waited an unreasonable length of time before being seen, nevertheless over 80% of these patients would opt for a specific appointment again. Less than a third of those who on their last visit had been given an open appointment would want the same sort of appointment again, and over two thirds of those who had had no appointments at all would, if given the choice, prefer a specific appointment time.

Table 7.12 Proportions of patients who on their last visit to hospital had been given a specific appointment time and who would prefer a specific appointment for future visits

For future visits would prefer . . .	On their last visit to hospital had:			All out-patients
	a specific appointment	an open appointment	no appoint-ment at all	
	%	%	%	%
a specific appointment	81	58	71	77
an open appointment	10	29	20	13
no preference	9	13	9	10
Base=all out-patients=100%	1648	179	435	2262

Analysis showed that there was no relationship between the time a patient had to wait to be seen on their last visit to hospital and the sort of appointment they would prefer for any future visits. However table 7.13 shows that patients who thought that waiting at least 15 minutes was unreasonable were marginally more likely to express a preference as to type of future appointment.

Table 7.13 Preference for future appointments analysed by attitude of patients waiting more than 15 minutes to be seen

For future visits would prefer . . .	Waiting about 15 minutes or longer on last visit was:	
	unreasonable	reasonable
	%	%
a specific appointment	80	75
an open appointment	16	14
no preference	4	11
Base=100%[1]	363	922

1. Base=all outpatients who on their last visit to hospital waited about 15 minutes or longer before being seen.

The type of appointment a patient prefers may, of course, be affected by their own domestic circumstances as much as by previous hospital experience. For example a working man may prefer the flexibility that an open appointment

Table 7.14 Proportions of men and women in different age groups who would prefer a specific appointment if they had to go to hospital again

For future visits patients would prefer . . .	Men aged:						All men	Women aged:						All women
	0–9	10–16	17–34	35–54	55–64	65 & over		0–9	10–16	17–34	35–54	55–64	65 & over	
	%	%	%	%	%	%	%	%	%	%	%	%	%	%
a specific appointment	79	77	73	79	78	74	77	80	74	79	82	80	72	78
an open appointment	18	16	19	11	10	6	13	14	17	18	12	11	6	13
no preference	3	7	8	10	12	20	10	6	9	3	6	9	22	9
Base: all outpatients=100%	160	135	280	257	154	169	1155	135	93	224	274	160	221	1107

allows, while an elderly person with fewer demands on their time may feel it matters less which type of appointment they are given.

Analysis showed that there was a clear preference by men of all ages for a specific appointment; between 74% and 79% of men in the various age groups would opt for this sort of appointment.

As can be seen from table 7.14 elderly men were more likely than younger men patients to say they had no preference as to type of appointment, and were correspondingly less likely to opt for an open appointment. The majority of women of all ages would also opt for a specific appointment, although, women aged 65 and over were much less likely to have a preference than younger women patients.

On closer inspection it was found that while much the same proportion of working and non-working men would opt for a specific appointment, a higher proportion of non-working men had no particular preference.

Women patients who had either full or part-time jobs were also more likely than other non-working women aged 16 and over to express a preference; for just under 90% of each group a specific appointment would be satisfactory, but while one in six working women would be satisfied with an open appointment, a higher ratio, one in four, of non-working women would prefer this sort of appointment.

Table 7.15   Proportions of working men and women who would prefer an open appointment if they had to go into hospital again

For future visits patients would prefer . . .	Men		All men aged 16 and over	Women		All women aged 16 and over
	working	not working		working	not working	
	%	%	%	%	%	%
a specific appointment	77	75	76	84	75	78
an open appointment	14	8	13	11	13	12
no preference	9	17	11	5	12	10
Base: all outpatients aged 16 and over=100%	601	277	878	364	518	882

Reasons for preferring specific appointment times

Patients who would prefer to be given an appointment for a specific time were asked why they would prefer this sort of appointment rather than an open appointment. Their answers are shown in the table below.

Two thirds of those who had opted for a specific appointment time had done so because they thought they were more likely to be seen quickly with a specific appointment than if they had an open appointment. It will be remembered that we found no evidence of this when looking at the last visit patients made to hospital (table 7.8 refers).

Table 7.16　Reasons for preferring a specific appointment to an open appointment

Reasons for preferring a specific appointment	%
More likely to be seen quickly	66
More convenient for making arrangements at work	18
Easier to organise domestic arrangements	8
Easier to organise travelling arrangements	6
Easier to plan rest of day (nothing else stated)	6
More convenient for hospital staff	8
Definite time acts as incentive to get there	17
Dislike waiting with other people	1
Other answers	3
Base: all outpatients who would prefer a specific appointment time=100%[1]	1738

1. Percentages add to more than 100 as some people gave more than one reason

Many patients said they preferred specific appointment times because they fitted in more easily with their own personal and domestic arrangements: they knew what time they would need to take off work, could plan their journeys to and from the hospital, and could make arrangements at home to suit their appointment time. However as shall be seen later many patients gave these same reasons in support of open appointments. About one in six of patients preferring specific appointment times said that a definite appointment acted as an incentive for them to get to hospital, and that they liked to have things organised and to know what was happening rather than to have a more vague arrangement. A small proportion felt that a specific appointment was helpful to the hospital staff, including ambulance drivers, as they knew how many patients to expect and would be ready for them, and this in turn helped to keep waiting times to a minimum, and about one in ten preferred specific appointment times because they disliked, or found it depressing, having to wait with other patients. Again there is an underlying assumption that open appointments lead to greater numbers of patients waiting to be seen at any one time, and hence to longer waiting times.

Reasons for preferring open appointments

The main reason given by patients for preferring an open appointment to having a specific appointment time, was that it allowed greater flexibility: 28% of patients opting for this sort of appointment said that it allowed them to decide when would be the most convenient time to attend hospital, and that if anything unexpected occurred they were not likely to miss or to have to cancel their appointment.

Many more patients obviously felt the same way, but were more explicit and pointed out particular ways in which such flexibility would be an advantage: for example, 17% of those opting for open appointments preferred them because they could attend at a time which fitted in most conveniently with their work, as one man said . . .

"If I could go (to hospital) at any time then I would go straight there and then on to work, and so save having to make two trips to work".

Table 7.17   Reasons for preferring an open appointment to a specific appointment time

Reasons for preferring an open appointment	%
Open appointment allows flexibility	28
More convenient for making arrangements at work	17
Easier to organise domestic arrangements	13
Easier to organise travelling arrangements	16
As good a chance of being seen quickly as with a specific appointment	24
Like freedom of choice (nothing else stated)	14
Other answers	4
Base: all outpatients who would prefer an open appointment=100%[1]	295

1. Percentages add to more than 100 as some people gave more than one reason.

It is difficult to see why an early specific appointment would not serve the same purpose.

One in eight of these patients, including the two quoted below, said open appointments were easier to fit in with their domestic circumstances . . .

"It's not always possible to manage a particular time with feeding the baby",

"It's easier for me to go when it suits me . . . when the children and my husband are on shift work",

and just over one in six felt they could avoid transport problems more easily if they had an open appointment. Several patients mentioned that as public transport was unreliable they had to leave home very early for specific appointments if they were to be certain of arriving on time at the hospital; with an open appointment this problem would not arise.[26]

It has already been seen that the most frequent reason given in support of specific appointment times was the greater chance of being seen quickly. Although patients preferring open appointments did not make this same claim, nevertheless one in four of these patients felt they had as good a chance of being seen quickly with an open appointment as with a specific appointment time. This together with the other advantages previously mentioned made them, on balance, favour open appointments.

7.5   The appointment system—for whose benefit?

As a further and final indication of opinions of the appointment system patients were asked the following question . . .

"And still thinking very generally, do you personally think that on the whole the hospital appointment system is mainly for the benefit of the doctors or mainly for the benefit of the patients?"

---

26. It has already been shown that one in four of all outpatients arriving early and one in six of all making their own way to hospital and arriving early for specific appointments, had no option as that was the time the transport arrived (see table 7.3).

Exactly half of all outpatients felt the system was mainly for the benefit of the doctors. The remainder were more or less equally divided into those who thought it was mainly for the benefit of the patients (24%) and those who, unprompted, said it was for the mutual and equal benefit of both doctors and patients—referred to as '50–50' in this discussion.

Although patients who had been given specific appointment times on their last visit to hospital were no more likely than those who had open appointments or no appointments at all to think that the system operated mainly for the benefit of doctors, those who did feel this was the way the system worked were more likely to opt for open appointments for any future visits to hospital if they were given the choice, than those who felt the appointment system was mainly for patients' benefit.

From what has been learnt already it was not surprising to find that the longer a patient had waited to be seen on their last visit to hospital the more likely they were to think that the appointment system was mainly for the benefit of the doctors. As can be seen from table 7.18 below while less than half of those who had to wait less than about 15 minutes to be seen on their last visit to hospital thought that the system was for the doctors' benefit, this proportion rose to nearly two thirds among those who had waited about an hour or even longer before being seen.

Table 7.18   Attitudes of patients waiting varying lengths of time to be seen as to who benefits by an appointment system

The appointment system is mainly for the benefit of . . .	Length of time patient waited before being seen					All out-patients[1]
	about 5–10 mins	about 15 mins	about 30 mins	about 45 mins	about 1 hour or longer	
	%	%	%	%	%	%
doctors	43	50	52	61	64	50
patients	28	25	22	17	18	24
'50–50'	29	25	26	22	18	26
Base: all outpatients=100%[1]	904	368	376	166	341	2155

1. excludes 13 patients who were either unconscious or had no idea of how long they waited

The impact of this last visit to hospital was demonstrated even more clearly by yet further analysis which showed that 70% of those who thought that waiting more than about 15 minutes to be seen was unreasonable, also thought that the system was mainly for the benefit of the doctors; 50% of those who had not minded waiting about 15 minutes or longer to be seen felt this way.

It has already been seen that older patients seem to be less critical of many aspects of the hospital service than younger men and women, and it has been suggested that this may, in part at least, be due to the different expectations that younger and older patients have. Here again there was evidence that older patients were less harsh in their judgement than younger patients: while about one in five patients aged under 35 thought the appointment system was mainly for the benefit of the patient, one in three of those aged 65 and over believed this to be so.

Table 7.19 **Proportion of patients in different age groups who thought the appointment system was mainly for the benefit of the doctors**

The appointment system is mainly for the benefit of . . .	Men and women aged						All out-patients
	0–9	10–16	17–34	35–54	55–64	65 & over	
	%	%	%	%	%	%	%
doctors	64	52	61	52	36	33	50
patients	14	24	18	22	35	35	24
'50–50'	22	24	21	26	29	32	26
Base: all out-patients=100%	290	221	492	510	305	375	2193

8.0   Privacy

In previous chapters it has been shown that some patients were dissatisfied because certain facilities or arrangements at the hospital afforded them insufficient privacy; for example 2% of adult inpatients spontaneously mentioned lack of privacy when washing and bathing. This chapter looks in more detail at patients' concern with privacy; complaints of lack of privacy when washing and bathing, or when visitors were there or when undressing for outpatient examinations or treatment are discussed, but the main part of this chapter reports patients' dissatisfaction with the amount of privacy they had during their consultation, examination or treatment, and to what extent this upset or disturbed them.

8.1   Privacy for inpatients

When washing and bathing

Although only 2% of all adult inpatients spontaneously mentioned that they were dissatisfied with the lack of privacy they had when washing and bathing, when specifically asked, 13% of all adult patients who had used these facilities while in hospital, felt there had been insufficient privacy.

Table 8.1: Proportion of men and women who had insufficient privacy when washing or bathing and who were bothered by it

Privacy when washing or bathing was . . .	Men	Women	Men and women
	%	%	%
adequate	88	87	87
inadequate and patient was:			
bothered quite a lot by it	2	5	4
bothered only a little	2	5	4
not really bothered at all	8	3	5
Base: all inpatients aged 14 and over using facilities=100%	233	447	680

Further analysis showed that although overall women were no more likely than men to have felt they had insufficient privacy when washing or bathing, they were more likely than men to be bothered by it.[27] One in ten adult women inpatients was bothered by insufficient privacy when washing or bathing compared with less than one in twenty adult men inpatients.

Insufficient privacy when visitors were there

The original data showed that lack of privacy during visiting sessions was a quite common experience; one in four adult patients who had had visitors while in hospital said that they personally had had insufficient privacy when their

---

27. Analysis showed that non-maternity women patients were more likely to have had inadequate privacy when washing or bathing than maternity patients, but the numbers involved were too small to compare how bothered these two groups were by this lack of privacy.

visitors were there. Somewhat surprisingly analysis showed that this was no more of a problem for patients in large wards than for those in smaller wards or rooms. However maternity patients were more likely to be dissatisfied than either other women patients or men patients, and analysis also showed that the younger patients were more likely to complain than older men and women (see tables 8.2 and 8.3).

Table 8.2: Proportions of men and women who did not have enough privacy when they had visitors

Privacy when visitors were there was . . .	Men	Women		Men and women
		maternity patients	non-maternity patients	
	%	%	%	%
adequate	80	65	79	77
inadequate	20	35	21	23
Base=100%[1]	242	97	360	699

1. Base=all inpatients aged 14 and over who had visitors while in hospital.

Table 8.3: Proportions of men and women patients in different age groups who did not have enough privacy when they had visitors

Patients who had visitors	Proportions who did not have enough privacy	Base=100%[1]
	%	
Men aged:		
14–34	31	58
35–54	19	80
55–64	23	48
65 and over	4	53
All men	19	239
Women aged:		
14–34	29	197
35–54	18	114
55–64	17	53
65 and over	16	83
All women	21	447

1. Base=all inpatients who had visitors.

Although lack of privacy during visiting sessions was a fairly frequent occurrence the majority of patients were not concerned by it; over half said that it had not really bothered them at all, and a further one in three said that they were only bothered a little by it. However the remaining 11% were bothered quite a lot by having inadequate privacy when their visitors were there.

Although the numbers involved were small there was some evidence to show that patients who were most likely to complain about lack of privacy for their visitors—maternity patients and younger patients—were also the groups most likely to be bothered by it. Over half of the maternity patients who had said there was inadequate privacy were bothered by it compared with about a third of other women patients, and 53% of patients between the ages of 14 and 34 were bothered by this lack of privacy compared with only 32% of those aged 35 and over.

Privacy during inpatient examinations and treatment

Nearly 90% of all adult inpatients felt that they had always had enough privacy when they were being treated or examined. Those who felt the privacy had always or even on some occasions been inadequate were asked whether, when they were being treated or examined, they could be overheard or seen by other patients.

The original data showed that the 12% of patients who did not have enough privacy included 11% who could be overheard by other patients during their examination, and 3% who could be seen by other patients. Overall 19 patients (3% of all adult inpatients) without adequate privacy said they could be both seen and overheard by other patients during their examinations or treatment. Further analysis (table 8.4 below) showed that patients in maternity wards were particularly likely to feel that they had had insufficient privacy and to say that they could be overheard during their examinations.

Table 8.4: Proportions of men and women patients who did not have enough privacy when being treated or examined and who could be overheard or seen by other patients during their examination or treatment

During examinations and treatment . . .	Men	Women		Men and women
		maternity patients	non-maternity patients	
	%	·%	%	%
always had enough privacy	89	78	89	88
did not have enough privacy:				
could be overheard	9	22	11	11
could be seen	2	3	3	3
Base: all inpatients aged 14 and over=100%[1]	241	97	357	695

1. percentages add to more than 100 as some patients could be seen and overheard

Not everyone may be concerned to the same extent about being seen or overheard during examination or treatment and indeed the data showed that just over 40% of those whose examinations could be heard by other patients were not bothered by this at all. However 23% of those being overheard said that it had bothered them quite a lot; not surprisingly, as many as 11 of the 19 patients who could be seen by other patients during their examinations were considerably bothered by this. The numbers involved were rather small but there was some indication that women were more likely to be concerned by lack of privacy than men.[28] By further analysis it was found that 24 patients (3% of all adult inpatients) were considerably disturbed because when they were being examined they could be *either* seen *or* overheard.

Although patients who were examined in view of other patients were more likely to be bothered by it than patients whose examinations could be overheard, overall the numbers of patients bothered by being overheard is greater than the number bothered by being seen. It would seem therefore, that for inpatients, being

---

28. Maternity patients seemed no more or less concerned that their examination could be overheard than other women patients.

96

overheard is more likely to contribute to a feeling of lack of privacy than being seen by other patients when being examined.

It may be of interest to compare the proportions who were concerned by lack of privacy during their examinations or treatment with the proportions concerned by lack of privacy when they had visitors and when washing or bathing. As can be seen from the table below being *seen* by other patients during an examination was most likely to cause distress, but more patients were bothered by lack of privacy when washing and bathing than by their examinations or treatment being overheard by other patients. Lack of privacy during visiting sessions gave rise to the least concern.

Table 8.5   Proportions of patients who were bothered by lack of privacy when washing or bathing, during visiting hours, and when being examined or treated

Patient was bothered by lack of privacy . . .	Lack of privacy when . . .			
	washing or bathing	visitors were there	being examined or treated	
			could be overheard	could be seen
	%	%	%	Nos
quite a lot	32	11	23	[11]
only a little	33	32	34	[3]
was not bothered	35	57	43	[5]
Base=100%[1]	88	145	79	19

1. Base=all adult patients who experienced lack of privacy.

Although the proportions of patients shown in the table as being bothered quite a lot by lack of privacy in these different situations vary considerably, it should be remembered that in each case the numbers represent less than 5% of all adult inpatients.

Although some people do not mind their own consultation or examination being overheard, they nevertheless find it embarrassing or upsetting to overhear what is being said to a fellow patient. Just over one in ten adult patients who did not have enough privacy during their examination or treatment found they could overhear what was being said to other patients, and about 40% were bothered to some extent by it. About 3% were able to see other patients being treated or examined and 12 of these 19 patients were bothered by this.[29]

8.2   Privacy for outpatients

When undressing

Just over half of all outpatients, on at least one occasion, had to undress to be treated or examined. Women in general, and in particular women aged between 35 and 54, were more likely to have had to undress than either men or women in other age groups.

---

29. Again although the numbers are small there was some indication that seeing or hearing other patients being treated or examined was more likely to upset women patients than men.

Table 8.6 Proportions of men and women in different age groups who had, on at least one occasion, to undress for treatment or examination

Outpatients	Patients who had to undress	Base=100%
	%	
Men aged:		
0–9	40	161
10–16	30	135
17–34	40	281
35–54	58	257
55–64	62	154
65 and over	61	170
All men	49	1158
Women aged:		
0–9	39	135
10–16	32	94
17–34	58	224
35–54	69	274
55–64	57	160
65 and over	57	222
All women	56	1109

Of the 1181 who did undress for examination or treatment 8% found the arrangements for undressing and getting dressed again unsatisfactory, the most common complaint, mentioned by over 40% of those who were dissatisfied, was that there was a lack of privacy. Closer inspection showed that women, who were more likely to have to undress anyway, were also more likely to be dissatisfied than men with the arrangements for getting changed, and that young women and young girls found the facilities unsatisfactory more often than older women patients.

Table 8.7 Proportions of men and women in different age groups who found the arrangements for undressing usually unsatisfactory

Outpatients who had to undress	Proportion who found arrangements unsatisfactory	Base=100%[1]
	%	
Men aged:		
0–9	9	64
10–16	[4]	41
17–34	9	111
35–54	9	148
55–64	7	95
65 and over	2	104
All men	7	563
Women aged:		
0–9	19	52
10–16	[8]	30
17–34	12	129
35–54	9	188
55–64	5	92
65 and over	5	127
All women	10	618

1. Base=all outpatients who had to undress for treatment or examination

98

As has already been mentioned, 43 of the 104 patients (41%) who were unhappy with the changing facilities said this was because there was insufficient privacy. These included patients who said there were no separate changing facilities at all—they had to undress in front of the doctor, that doors to cubicles were left open, or had no locks, and that curtains failed to close properly. One in eight of these patients complained that there was nowhere to hang their clothes, they had to be left on the floor or on a chair, and one in ten were worried by the lack of security for their personal possessions—there were no lockers and they had to leave their things behind in a cubicle which would be used by other patients. Small numbers of patients complained about the gowns; none were provided, they were too small, or they had no ties, and that they were asked to undress too long before their examination or treatment. Several mothers who had to undress young babies said they would have found a table that they could have laid the baby on helpful.

Privacy during outpatient consultations, examinations and treatment

One in four of all outpatients said that on their last visit to hospital, when they went in for their consultation, examination or their treatment, other patients who were also being attended to or who were waiting to be seen could overhear what was being said to them. Two thirds of all outpatients were certain they could not be overheard, and for 146 there had been no possibility of such a situation arising as they had been the only patient there at the time. The original data also showed that one in seven patients were treated, examined or had their consultation in view of other patients and analysis showed that 209 patients (10%) could be *both* seen *and* overheard.

As can be seen from the table below lack of privacy during examination was experienced most often by patients attending physiotherapy, casualty, and ophthalmic or dental clinics.

Table 8.8   Proportion of patients attending various outpatient departments who could be overheard or be seen by other patients during their consultation, examination or treatment

Department or clinic attended		Proportion of patients who could be . . .			Base=100%[1]
		overheard by other patients	seen by other patients	overheard *and* seen	
physiotherapy	%	62	24	20	50
casualty	%	46	24	18	427
ophthalmic or dental	%	31	30	23	117
orthopaedic	%	38	7	5	55
outpatients	%	21	10	7	975
X-ray	%	19	5	1	104
gynaecology	%	17	—	—	48
ENT	%	12	7	5	42
paediatric	nos	[2]	[1]	[—]	27
others	%	22	12	8	273
all outpatients	%	28	14	10	2118

1. base excludes those who were the only patient in the clinic at that time

Further analysis (table 8.9) also showed that patients aged between 17 and 34, and those accompanying babies and young children, were most likely to complain that they could be overheard or seen by other patients. Men were also more likely than women to have been treated or examined in view of other patients; about one in six men said they could be seen by other patients compared to about one in eight women.

Table 8.9   Proportions of men and women who could be overheard or seen by other patients during their consultation, examination, or treatment

Outpatients	Proportion who could be		Base=100%[1]
	overheard	seen	
	%	%	
Men and women aged:			
0–9	36	21	269
10–16	27	15	212
17–34	38	17	455
35–54	30	11	487
55–64	20	11	299
65 and over	16	9	361
All men	28	16	1060
All women	28	12	1023
All men and women	28	14	2083

1. base excludes those who were the only patient in the clinic at that time

As was found for inpatients, the majority of outpatients whose consultation, examination, or treatment could be overheard by other patients were not bothered at all by this; the original data showed that 85% were not bothered at all, 9% were bothered only a little and that only 6% were bothered quite a lot by being overheard. However being treated within view of other patients was for outpatients, unlike inpatients, no more likely to cause concern than being overheard: 82% of outpatients who could be seen by other patients when being treated said that this had not bothered them at all, the remainder were equally divided into those who were bothered quite a lot, and those concerned only a little.

It can be seen from table 8.10 that women aged between 17 and 34 were most likely to be concerned that their consultation, examination or treatment could be overheard and that men were equally as likely as women to be concerned at being examined in view of other patients. However nearly one in four patients aged between 17 and 34 who were examined in view of other patients were bothered by this, and those taking babies and young children under the age of ten to hospital were also more likely to be upset by this lack of privacy than other patients.

About one in four outpatients said that when they were at the hospital they sometimes found they could hear what was being said to other patients, and 111 of these 524 patients (21%) said that this had bothered them. A much smaller proportion (about one in eight) said they were able to see other patients being examined or treated, and of these, 18% said they were bothered by this lack of privacy. As can be seen from table 8.11 women were far more likely than men to be upset by overhearing doctors' consultations with other patients, but men were just as likely as women to be bothered by seeing other patients being examined or treated. Analysis also showed that younger patients, and those accompanying babies and young children to hospital were more likely to be bothered than older patients by this lack of privacy for other patients.

Table 8.10: Proportions of men and women who were bothered by being overheard or seen by other patients during their consultation, examination or treatment

Patient was bothered by lack of privacy . . .	Patients whose consultation, examination or treatment could be . . .																				
	overheard by other patients											seen by other patients								
	Men aged				All men	Women aged				All women	All men and women	Men and women aged					All men	All women	All men and women
	0-16	17-34	35-54	55 & over		0-16	17-34	35-54	55 & over			0-9	10-16	17-34	35-54	55 & over			
	%	%	%	%	%	%	%	%	%	%	%	%	Nos	%	%	%	%	%	%
quite a lot	4	4	8	2	4	8	10	4	9	8	6	14	[1]	11	9	3	7	11	8
only a little	1	3	5	6	4	11	29	13	6	15	9	14	[1]	12	7	4	7	11	9
was not bothered	95	93	87	92	92	81	61	83	85	77	85	72	[30]	77	84	93	86	78	83
Base=100%¹	83	96	74	48	301	72	77	70	69	288	589	57	32	81	55	68	171	122	293

1. base=all who experienced lack of privacy

Table 8.11 Proportion of men and women patients and patients in different age groups who were bothered by overhearing or seeing other patients being consulted, examined or treated

Outpatients	Bothered by overhearing other patients being treated etc.		Bothered by seeing other patients being treated etc.	
	%	Base=100%[1]	%	Base=100%[2]
Men and women aged:				
0–9	21	77	}20	}76
10–16	[8]	47		
17–34	29	165	28	72
35–54	22	135	[5]	44
55 and over	11	100	8	63
All men	15	269	18	146
All women	28	255	17	109
All men and women	21	524	18	255

1. base=all outpatients who could overhear other patients being consulted, examined or treated.
2. base=all outpatients who could see other patients being consulted, examined or treated.

8.3 Summary

In this chapter it has been shown that although lack of privacy is experienced by many patients, not all patients are concerned or bothered by it.

One in ten adult inpatients who, overall, had not had enough privacy during their examinations or treatment could be overheard by other patients, and 3% were examined or treated in view of other patients. Just over one in four of *all* outpatients could, during their consultation, examination or treatment be overheard by other patients, and 14% said they could be seen by other patients when they were being treated or examined. Many of those who had experienced this lack of privacy had been bothered by it and inpatients in particular seemed concerned at being seen by others: 14 of the 19 inpatients who overall had not had enough privacy and whose examinations were visible to other patients were bothered by this, compared to 17% of all outpatients who could be seen when examined or treated. These proportions represent 2% of all adult inpatients and 2% of all outpatients. Just under one in four adult inpatients with insufficient privacy and whose examinations could be overheard by other patients were bothered quite a lot by it (representing 3% of all adult inpatients) compared to 6% of outpatients whose examinations were within other patients' hearing (2% of all outpatients). Analysis has shown that generally it is women and the younger outpatients who are most likely to be distressed by this lack of privacy.

Seeing and overhearing other patients being examined or treated was as frequent an occurrence as being seen or overheard by others, and the data showed that although generally it bothered fewer people it still upset a considerable number of patients. The only exception found to this was outpatients who were more likely to be upset by overhearing other patients' consultations, than by being overheard themselves.

9.0 Communication

Going into hospital, or attending hospital as an outpatient is for many patients an extremely anxious time and to relieve at least some of this anxiety the patient must have confidence in those who are caring for them. That the very best medical treatment and care is being provided may do little to allay any anxiety if the patient feels he is not being given enough information about his condition, treatment and progress. Of course, what one patient regards as adequate information may be inadequate for another, indeed some patients prefer to be told as little as possible, and there is an additional problem for the doctors and nurses in that not all patients are able to grasp and understand the information given to them.

There is an opportunity for many inpatients at a very early stage to be provided with a booklet or leaflet giving some general information about the way the hospital is organised, its facilities and about what they can expect to be the routine once they are in hospital. This chapter starts by looking at the extent of provision of such booklets and at how useful inpatients find them, and then goes on to consider the problems some patients (both inpatients and outpatients) have in obtaining and understanding information about their condition, treatment and progress.

9.1 The information booklet for inpatients

The original data show that 40% of all inpatients were given an explanatory booklet or leaflet about the hospital before they were admitted, and a further 19% were given it on admission or soon after.

Nearly all (95%) of the 470 inpatients who had been given a booklet or leaflet explaining about the hospital and its facilities found it useful, and 54% said it had been very useful to them. The two main complaints from patients who had not found it of any use were firstly, that the booklet did not contain enough information, it was generally restricted to details of visiting arrangements and telephone numbers, and secondly, and this applied particularly to visiting hours, that the information it contained was incorrect or out-of-date.

The most popular points that patients would have liked included in the booklet were more information about facilities—shops, dayrooms, etc, and the parents of children going into hospital would have liked to have known whether they should take their child's own clothes and toys to the hospital with them.

9.2 Communication between doctors and inpatients

Being given insufficient information about treatment and progress

The original data show that nearly one in three patients felt that they had not been given enough information about how they were progressing. This includes the parents of child patients and maternity patients who felt they were not being told enough about how their children or babies were getting on. Indeed, further analysis showed that parents whose young children were in hospital were particularly likely to feel they were getting insufficient information, and that young men and women patients between the ages of 17 and 34 were also more likely than older patients to want to know more. Only about half of these younger patients felt they had been given enough information (table 9.1 below).

Table 9.1 Proportions of men and women in different age groups who felt they were not told enough about how they (or their child or baby) were progressing

All inpatients aged:	Proportion who were not told enough and wanted to know more[1]	Base=100%
	%	
0–9	37	79
10–16	21	29
17–34	43	249
35–54	30	196
55–64	23	102
65 and over	17	136
All male inpatients	31	307
All female inpatients	31	484
All inpatients	31	791

1. Patients who did not want to know how they were progressing were regarded as having been told enough.

Not being told very much about how one is progressing may not be a problem if it is possible to ask the doctors what one wants to know, and then to get a satisfactory answer to the questions one asks. Nearly half (47%) of the patients (or parents) who wanted more information felt they could not ask any of their doctors to tell them what they wanted to know, and a further 15% felt they could ask only some of their doctors. Thus nearly one in seven of all the inpatients interviewed had been given what they felt was insufficient information about their progress, and felt unable to ask any of the doctors to tell them what they wanted to know.

That some patients felt they could not approach some of the doctors does not necessarily reflect badly on the doctors' attitude; many people are timid or shy of talking to people in what they regard as authority; they feel it is not their place to ask questions. However when asked why they felt unable to ask questions only six out of 113 patients (5%) said that it was because they felt shy or nervous: they made no mention of finding the doctors' manner abrupt or intimidating in any way. A further 15 patients (13%) could give no explanation as to why they felt this way or why they had not asked for more information. The two most frequently given reasons for feeling unable to ask questions were the doctors seemed so busy and were in too much of a hurry to have time to answer questions (mentioned by 28% of the 113 patients) and the patients were deterred from asking by the doctors' attitude—mentioned by 27% of these patients. These 31 patients said they found the doctors' manner very abrupt, they felt the doctors regarded them as being incapable of understanding their explanations, or they were very offhand and gave the impression that it was not the patient's place to ask questions. Just under one in five patients feeling unable to ask questions said that lack of opportunity was the problem; comments such as these were made...

"no doctors visited towards the end of my stay when I wanted to ask questions",

and from the parents of young children . . .

"the doctors were never available if you wanted to see them, and the nurses wouldn't arrange for you to see them" and

"we didn't see the doctor. We only saw him when he (child) was ready for discharge".

Small numbers of patients felt there was no point in asking questions, because the doctors evaded their questions and they never got what they felt were satisfactory answers, or because the doctors were foreign and they could not understand them, or because the answers they got were given in terms they could not understand. All inpatients were specifically asked about these three points later in the interview and the findings are discussed in this chapter.

Although the majority of patients who felt they could ask at least some of their doctors to tell them what they wanted to know said that they generally got a satisfactory answer to the questions they asked, nevertheless 30% said their questions were not generally answered to their satisfaction. Although the numbers involved are small there was some indication that elderly patients were most likely to be satisfied.

The table below summarises patients' satisfaction with the communication that passed between themselves and their doctors as to how they were progressing.

Table 9.2   Proportions of patients who were able to get sufficient information about how they were progressing from their doctors

Patients who were . . .	%	
Always told enough about how progressing	71	
Not told enough, wanted to know more and . . .		82%
could ask all or some doctors and got a satisfactory answer	11	
could ask all doctors but did not get a satisfactory answer	4	
could not ask any doctors	14	18%
Base: all inpatients=100%	780	

It can be seen that over 80% of patients were satisfied either because they were adequately informed about how they were progressing, or because they could ask questions and get satisfactory answers, but nearly one in five inpatients (18%) were dissatisfied because they were unable to get sufficient information on how they were getting on.

Difficulties in understanding

Despite the fact that a patient may be told how he is progressing, or be able to get satisfactory answers to the questions he asks, the information he is given at any time during his stay in hospital may not be of very much use if he is unable to understand what he is being told. It has already been seen that there are two dimensions to this problem: a patient may not understand if medical terminology is used when explaining about his condition or treatment, or he may have difficulty in understanding if either he, or the doctor, is foreign and has poorly spoken English or a strong accent. One in four patients had difficulty with medical terminology and would have liked to have been told about their condition or treatment in 'everyday language', and about one in seven patients had problems, apart from this, in simply understanding what the doctor was saying.[30] In a small number of cases this was because the patient was hard of hearing or was foreign and had difficulty in understanding English, but one in eight patients specifically mentioned that their difficulty was in understanding foreign doctors.

Analysis showed that elderly patients were the least likely to have had difficulty with medical terminology which suggests that doctors are making a particular effort with elderly patients to explain things to them in everyday language. However as can be seen from table 9.3 more than one in three patients aged between 17 and 34 experienced this problem.

Table 9.3   **Proportions of men and women patients in different age groups who had difficulty in understanding what the doctors told them about their condition or treatment**

All inpatients aged:	Proportions of patients who had difficulty in understanding . . .		Base=100%
	because medical terms were used	for other reasons, mainly because doctors were foreign	
	%	%	
0–16	21	11	107
17–34	36	20	249
35–54	26	15	193
55–64	22	14	102
65 and over	10	10	135
All male inpatients	24	10	306
All female inpatients	25	18	480
All inpatients	25	15	786

Problems in simply understanding the doctors apart from their using medical terminology were generally as likely to have been experienced by older patients as by younger patients, although female patients and patients aged between 17 and 34 appeared to find it a problem somewhat more often than other patients.[31]

Having difficulty in understanding what a doctor is saying may affect different patients in different ways; some may not bother about it, others may be prepared to ask another doctor or nurse to explain in everyday language what they had not understood (just under half—49%—of those having difficulty with medical terminology did ask someone else to explain) while others may feel embarrassed or worried and upset at not understanding.

30. 47 patients (6%) experienced both sorts of problem.

31. The high proportion of patients aged between 17 and 34 having difficulty was largely accounted for by the large number of women in this group: 45 of the 200 (23%) women aged 17 to 34 had difficulty compared with 5 of the 49 men (10%).

The original data show that nearly half the 288 patients who did not understand what their doctors told them about their condition or treatment because they used medical terminology, or for any other reason, were not really bothered by it, but that 28% were worried or upset at not understanding, and 26% were embarrassed by it. A small number of patients were both worried and embarrassed.

By analysis (table 9.4) it was found that men and patients aged 55 and over were significantly less likely to be bothered by not understanding than women and younger patients. Patients aged between 17 and 34 whom it has been shown were most likely both to want to know more about how they were progressing and to have difficulty in understanding, were also the most likely to worry or be embarrassed about not understanding.

Table 9.4 Proportions of men and women aged 17 and over[1] worried or embarrassed by not understanding what the doctors told them about their condition or treatment

Attitude to not understanding	All inpatients aged:			All aged 17 and over		
	17–34	35–54	55 and over	Men	Women	Men and women
	%	%	%	%	%	%
not really bothered	31	63	72	68	41	49
worried or upset	32	29	16	19	31	28
embarrassed	38	12	12	14	30	25
Base=100%[2][3]	103	51	49	59	144	203

1. As there were only 25 patients aged between 0–16 they have been excluded from this table.
2. Base=all inpatients who could not understand what the doctors told them about their condition or treatment.
3. Percentages add to more than 100 as some people were both worried and embarrassed.

9.3 Communication between doctors and outpatients

All outpatients interviewed were asked the same series of questions as inpatients about how satisfied they were with the amount of information they had been given by the doctors, whether they felt able to ask for more information and whether they had any difficulties in understanding the doctors.

Being given insufficient information about treatment and progress

Three out of four outpatients said that the doctors they had seen at the hospital had always told them enough about how they were getting on, and analysis showed that young patients between the ages of 17 and 34 were most likely to have felt they wanted to know more. As can be seen from the table below nearly one in three patients aged 17 to 34 wanted more information about how they were progressing compared to about one in four of other patients.

It was not surprising also to find that one in five outpatients who had made only one visit to hospital for that condition wanted to know more, while a significantly greater proportion, one in four, of those who had made more than one visit, felt they wanted more information on how they were progressing.

Table 9.5 Proportion of outpatients in different age groups who wanted to know more about how they were getting on

All outpatients aged:	Proportion who were not told enough and wanted to know more[1]	Base=100%[2]
	%	
0–9	27	294
10–16	21	229
17–34	31	497
35–54	26	524
55–64	24	309
65 and over	21	388
All male outpatients	24	1142
All female outpatients	27	1099
All outpatients	25	2241

1. Patients who did not want to know how they were progressing were regarded as having been told enough.
2. Base=all outpatients, excluding those who did not regard the person they saw as a doctor.

It was found, as with inpatients, that a large proportion (42%) of the 567 outpatients who wanted more information felt unable to ask any of the doctors to tell them what they wanted to know, and that a further 13% felt they could only ask some doctors. For the larger outpatient sample it was possible to carry out further analysis.

Table 9.6 Proportions of men and women in different age groups who felt unable to ask the doctors to tell them what they wanted to know

Those who wanted to know more about how they were progressing and . . .	All outpatients aged:					All men	All women	All out-patients
	0–16	17–34	35–54	55–64	65 & over			
	%	%	%	%	%	%	%	%
could ask *all* doctors	37	42	45	51	58	50	40	45
could ask only *some* doctors	8	9	20	21	7	10	15	13
could not ask *any* doctors	55	49	35	28	35	40	45	42
Base: all outpatients who wanted to know more about how they were progressing =100%	126	153	132	75	81	276	291	567

This showed, as can be seen from table 9.6, that although the proportions of men and women patients who felt unable to ask *any* of the doctors to tell them what they wanted to know were similar, men were more likely than women to feel able to approach any doctor at all. The analysis also shows that younger patients and especially the parents of young children attending hospital as outpatients, were particularly likely to feel unable to ask any doctor to tell them what they wanted to know about their, or their child's condition or treatment.

The main reason for feeling unable to ask any of the doctors for more information was that their manner was abrupt or in some other way off-putting; 43% of those patients who felt they could not ask any of the doctors to tell them what they wanted to know, gave this reason and a similar proportion (40%) felt unable to ask because the doctors seemed in too much of a hurry or too busy to deal with their questions. While one in ten of these patients said they themselves were too shy or too nervous to ask questions, an equal number did not bother to ask as they felt they would not have got a satisfactory answer or have been told anything more. One in seven could give no reason as to why they felt unable to ask for more information about their condition or treatment. As was found for inpatients, small numbers of outpatients had not asked the doctors to tell them what they wanted to know either because the doctors used terminology they could not understand, or because they were foreign, and it was difficult to understand their English.

Although the majority of patients who asked for more information said they generally got satisfactory answers, the proportion dissatisfied with the answers they got (40%) is nevertheless considerable. There was however no evidence that men rather than women, or that patients in any particular age group were more likely to have generally got satisfactory answers to their questions than any other group.

From the summary table below it can be seen that over 80% of outpatients were satisfied either because they were told all they wanted to know about how they were getting on, or because they felt able to ask at least some of the doctors and when they did so, they usually got a satisfactory answer.

Table 9.7   Proportion of outpatients who were able to get sufficient information about how they were progressing

Patients who were . . .	%	
Always told enough about how progressing	75	
Not told enough, wanted to know more and . . .		83%
could ask all or some doctors and got a satisfactory answer	8	
could ask all or some doctors but did not get a satisfactory answer	6	17%
could not ask any doctors	11	
Base: all outpatients=100%	2218	

However one in six outpatients were unable to get as much information as they would have liked about their condition, treatment and progress.

Difficulties in understanding

The original data show that 15% of outpatients had difficulty in understanding what the doctors told them about their condition and treatment: the doctors had used medical terminology and these patients would have liked to have had an explanation in everyday language. A similar proportion said that apart from the doctors using medical terms, they had trouble in simply understanding what some of the doctors were saying.[32] A small proportion of these patients said the trouble was due to their being hard of hearing, a few said that the doctors did not speak very clearly, they mumbled or muttered, and some patients had difficulty themselves in understanding English, but overall 13% of outpatients had difficulty in understanding what was being said to them because their doctors were foreign.

As was shown for inpatients, doctors would seem to be taking more care to explain about examinations and treatment in everyday language to elderly patients than to younger outpatients. Only 8% of outpatients aged 65 and over said they had difficulty in understanding and would have liked a more simple explanation, compared with about 16% of all other patients (see table 9.8 below).

Table 9.8   Proportions of men and women outpatients in different age groups who had difficulty
in understanding what the doctors told them about their condition or treatment

Outpatients	Proportions of patients who had difficulty in understanding . . .		Base=100%[1]
	because medical terms were used	for other reasons, mainly because doctors were foreign	
	%	%	
All outpatients aged:			
0–9	17	20	292
10–16	19	16	228
17–34	16	19	492
35–54	16	16	520
55–64	12	10	306
65 and over	8	10	383
All male outpatients	13	14	1133
All female outpatients	16	17	1088
All outpatients	15	15	2221

1. excludes those who did not regard the person they saw as a doctor

Female patients seemed generally to encounter more difficulty than men; they were both more likely to want things explained in everyday language than men, and were also more likely to have had other sorts of problems in understanding what the doctors were saying. Elderly patients in addition to being less likely to have difficulty in understanding the explanations they were given were also found to have fewer problems in simply understanding what the doctors were saying.[33] However patients aged between 17 and 34 and the parents of young children attending as outpatients were the most likely to experience these difficulties; one in five of those accompanying babies and young children under the age of ten to hospital for outpatient treatment said they had problems in simply understanding what the doctors were saying, apart from any difficulty they might have had in understanding medical terminology.

32. 109 outpatients (5%) experienced both sorts of problem.

33. Analysis showed that the small proportion of patients aged 65 and over who had difficulty in understanding was not accounted for by differences in the proportions of men and women in this group, but was a true function of age.

110

Of the 324 outpatients who would have liked to have been told about their condition or treatment in everyday language, 118 (36%) had asked another doctor or nurse to explain what had been said to them. However, of the 483 patients who for any reason had difficulty in understanding what the doctors said to them, 161 (33%) were worried or upset by not understanding, 25% of patients were embarrassed by it, and 42% said they were not bothered. By analysis (table 9.9) it was found that men outpatients and patients aged 65 and over were significantly less likely to be bothered by not understanding than women and younger patients (the groups most likely to encounter problems of this sort). Patients aged 55 and over were marginally less likely than younger patients to be worried or upset by not understanding what the doctor told them, and considerably less embarrassed than other patients by it.[34]

Table 9.9   **Proportions of men and women in different age groups worried or embarrassed by not understanding what the doctors told them about their condition or treatment**

Attitude to not understanding . . .	All outpatients aged:				All men	All women	All out-patients
	0–16	17–34	35–54	55 & over			
	%	%	%	%	%	%	%
not really bothered	28	42	45	58	48	37	42
worried or upset	35	33	33	31	30	36	33
embarrassed	38	26	23	10	22	28	25
Base=100%[1] [2]	133	129	116	105	227	256	483

1. Base=all outpatients who could not understand what the doctors told them about their condition or treatment.
2. Percentages add to more than 100 as some people were both worried and embarrassed.

34. Again this was checked and found to be a genuine function of age and not due to the sex composition of the group: although women generally were more likely to be bothered by not understanding, of the 61 women aged 55 and over, 37 were not bothered and six were embarrassed by it and of the 44 men in this age group, 24 were not bothered and 5 embarrassed by not understanding.

10.0 Relationships between patients and hospital staff

In the previous chapter the importance of adequate communications between doctor and patient in allaying anxiety and helping increase the patients' confidence was commented upon. Good relationships generally between the staff and patients will help the patient adjust more easily and quickly to being in hospital, and may even help them accept treatment more readily. However situations involving the staff and patients which cause the patient embarrassment or distress will undoubtedly affect a patient's attitude to treatment. This may happen if, for example, the patient is apparently ignored or excluded from discussions, or if they feel they are being treated as an exhibit rather than an individual, perhaps because students are present. These points and the patients' general views on the staff they met while they were in or attending hospital are discussed in this chapter.

10.1 The views of inpatients

The presence of medical students

Both as a common courtesy and to help avoid the patient feeling like an object on display, it is official DHSS policy that patients' permission should be obtained if medical students are to be present during a consultation or during treatment. Not all patients were asked whether their permission had been sought, nor whether they had any objections to medical students being present. These questions were limited to those who said they had insufficient privacy when being examined or treated.

The 88 inpatients aged 14 and over who felt they had generally had insufficient privacy when being examined or treated, were asked whether medical students had been present on any occasion when they were being examined or treated. Just under half (49%) had been examined or treated while students were there and of these 43 patients, 31 said they did not remember being asked whether they agreed to the students being present. However, the data show that the majority of these 31 patients were neither bothered by not being asked, nor had they minded the medical students being there. Seven patients were disturbed at not being asked and five of these seven patients also objected to the students' presence.

Being disregarded or ignored

One in four adult inpatients said that the doctors had discussed their condition or treatment with other people *as if they weren't there*. Apart from making the patients feel ignored and having no control over what is happening to them, it may have the more serious consequence of making them feel some unpleasant truth is being kept from them. In fact just under half the 171 patients who felt excluded in this way, were not bothered by it. However 55% (representing 13% of all inpatients aged 14 and over) said that they were annoyed, distressed or in some other way unhappy about this having happened. Their comments included the following. . . .

> "*I think it's terrible. You weren't supposed to hear but you could. I didn't think it was fair, you don't know if they are talking about you or not, you start thinking you have all sorts of things wrong with you they haven't told you about*".

> "*I thought it was a cheek, almost like a lump of meat, no feeling or interest in what was happening to you*".

> "*Annoyed. They sort of turn their backs on you*".

Although the numbers involved are small, there was some evidence to show that for any age group women were more likely to be distressed or annoyed at being treated in this way than men, while older patients, both men and women, were more likely than younger patients not to bother or take any notice of doctors discussing their condition or treatment with other people as if they were not there.

Table 10.1 Men and women inpatients aged 14 and over who were annoyed or distressed by doctors discussing them as if they were not there

All inpatients aged:	Proportions annoyed or distressed	Base=100%[1]
	%	
14–34	66	76
35–54	56	50
55 and over	[16]	45
All men aged 14 and over	41	65
All women aged 14 and over	63	106
All inpatients aged 14 and over	55	171

1. base=all inpatients whose condition or treatment was discussed as if they were not there

Relationships in general with the hospital staff

All inpatients (and the parents of young children who had been in hospital) were asked what proportion ("*all, most, or only a few*") of the nursing staff they met while they were in hospital "*were considerate*", what proportion of the para-medical staff (radiographers, physiotherapists, dieticians etc) were "*nice to them*", and what proportion of the non-medical staff (porters, orderlies etc) were "*helpful*". Some patients had not met some of these people while they were in hospital or felt they had met too few to comment and they have been excluded from the analyses. The original data show (table 10.2 below) that the vast majority of patients found that all or most of the staff in the three groups defined were considerate, or nice, or helpful.

No more than 5% of patients were dissatisfied with the majority of staff in any of the three groups, and it should be remembered that there are over-demanding patients as well as off-hand staff.

Table 10.2   Proportions of inpatients who were satisfied with the attitude of various groups of hospital staff they met while in hospital

Proportions of staff who were considerate, nice or helpful	Attitude of hospital staff		
	nursing staff who were considerate	para-medical staff who were nice to patients[1]	non-medical staff who were helpful
	%	%	%
all	64	86	80
most	31	12	16
only a few	5	2	4
Base=100%[2]	793	609	726

1. Physiotherapists, radiographers, dieticians etc.
2. Base=all inpatients who met sufficient staff to be able to comment

Relationships between hospital staff and child patients

The parents of child patients (children under 14) were asked whether they thought the staff had done all they could to reassure and comfort their child. Of the 98 parents, just under one in four (23%) were dissatisfied and felt the staff could have done more. The majority of these parents were concerned because they felt their child had been left alone too long; some parents felt their children got bored and lonely and that the staff should have spent more time with them, talking and playing with them individually, but a small number of parents (five) specifically complained (not saying how they knew) that their children were left crying for long periods with no-one to comfort them. Having someone with the child to reassure them when they came round from an anaesthetic, making more effort to explain about an operation and an anaesthetic, and having more supervision on the ward were further suggestions each put forward by two parents.

Helping patients adapt to being in hospital

So far we have concentrated on the relationship between hospital staff and patients. There are however many other people with whom the patient may have had contact while in hospital, for example, other patients, voluntary helpers, and their own visitors, all of whom may have helped them adapt to being in hospital and been able to reassure them about their condition and treatment. Indeed it has already been noted that one of the reasons given in favour of large wards was the mutual support and help that patients can give each other. Patients (and the parents of child patients) were asked who, of all the people they came into contact with while they were there, did most to help them adapt to being in hospital.

Over two thirds (67%) of all inpatients (including the parents of child patients) felt the nursing staff had done most to help them adapt to their stay in hospital, this includes 17% who specifically mentioned the ward sister as being particularly helpful in this respect. Other patients in the same ward as the patient had fulfilled this role for 10% of inpatients, although women were more likely to have found other patients helpful than men; only 6% of men thought other patients had done most to help them adapt compared to 13% of women. A small proportion of patients (6%) thought the hospital doctors had done most to help them settle down but 5% felt they could not pick out any one person or group of people as having done more than anyone else. Included in the group of miscellaneous answers (9%) were patients who felt they themselves had been mainly responsible for their adapting to life in hospital, those who thought their own GP the most helpful person, parents who felt they had done most in this respect for their own children, and patients who mentioned various other hospital workers such as cleaners, tea ladies, porters, and the voluntary helpers. One man felt that the information booklet provided by the hospital had done most to help him adapt to his stay in hospital.

Table 10.3   Who did most to help the patient adapt to being in hospital

Who did most to help patient adapt . . .	Men	Women	Men and Women
	%	%	%
nursing staff:			
ward sister	20	16	17
other nursing staff	47	51	50
other patients	6	13	10
hospital doctors	8	5	6
patients' relatives	2	2	2
everybody—could not choose	5	5	5
other answers	12	8	10
Base: all inpatients=100%	305	487	792

Being treated as an individual

At the conclusion of this section patients (and parents) were asked whether, on the whole, they felt they (or their child) had been treated as an individual or as just another case.

It has already been seen that one in four adult inpatients said their condition was discussed by doctors *as if they weren't there*, and at this question, which attempted to summarise how patients felt about their relationships with the medical staff, the data show that overall more than one in three felt they, or their child, had been treated as *just another case*.

Table 10.4   Proportions of patients in different age groups who, on the whole, felt they had been treated as just another case

On the whole patient was treated . . .	Patients aged:					All in-patients
	0–16	17–34	35–54	55–64	65 & over	
	%	%	%	%	%	%
as an individual	66	49	66	76	76	64
just another case	34	51	34	24	24	36
Base: all inpatients=100%	109	249	195	102	137	792

As can be seen from the table above, this lack of recognition as an individual was felt most keenly by patients aged between 17 and 34, over half of whom felt they were just another patient; in contrast 76% of older patients aged 55 and over felt they had been treated as an individual. Whether doctors and nurses genuinely behave differently towards more elderly patients, or whether elderly patients themselves have a different perception is difficult to tell, but it has already been noted that doctors appear to take more trouble to explain things to elderly patients in everyday language than they do with younger patients (table 9.3 refers). Contrary to many of the other findings of this study, it was found that women in general, and even maternity patients were no more likely to be dissatisfied with this aspect of their treatment than men, and hence the differences between the different age groups are not reflecting any differences in the sex composition of the groups.

On checking, it was also found that a high proportion (30 out of 37) of patients who had spent their entire stay in hospital in a room on their own, not unexpectedly, felt they had been treated as an individual. For those who had spent at least some time in a ward with other patients there was no relationship between the size of ward and the likelihood of feeling that one had been treated as just another case.

10.2 The views of outpatients on relationships between themselves and the hospital staff

A more limited range of questions on this topic was put to outpatients; they were asked only about how they felt about the presence of medical students and about how considerate, nice or helpful they found some of the hospital staff.

The presence of medical students

Just under one in four (23%) of all outpatients were examined or treated in the presence of medical students on at least one of their visits to hospital, but of these 514 patients only 169 (33%) remembered ever being asked if they agreed to the students being present, and a further 15 could not remember whether or not their permission was sought.

However of the 330 outpatients who were certain they had not been asked, 15% objected to not being asked; the majority were not really bothered that their permission had not been sought for students to be present. Yet again, analysis showed that for each age group women patients were more likely than men to object to not being asked, and among both men and women those aged 55 and over were considerably less likely to be bothered than either younger patients or the parents of child patients. While nearly one in five women who had not been asked whether they agreed to students being present, objected to not being asked, only about one in ten men objected, and while less than 5% of both men and women aged 65 and over were bothered that their permission had not been sought, the corresponding proportion for those aged between 17 and 34 was 22%.

Although patients might resent not being asked, they would not necessarily have objected to the presence of the students. Overall 32 outpatients (including eight parents) objected to the presence of medical students; this represents 6% of those who were examined or treated with students there and 10% of those whose permission was not sought.[35] The same pattern as had previously been seen, was found in further analysis of this data: women of all ages and particularly those aged between 17 and 34 were more likely to be worried by students being present than men patients.

Table 10.5   Summary table showing outpatients' attitudes to the presence of medical students (those who remembered whether their permission had been sought)

Patients' attitudes to medical students	%
No medical students present	78
Medical students present and . . .	
patient's permission sought	8
patient's permission not sought but . . .	
did not object to students' presence	13
objected to students' presence	1
Base=100%	2248

Relationships in general with the hospital staff

As was found for the inpatient sample the majority of outpatients also held most of the staff they had met during their visits to hospital in high regard, although obviously a much greater proportion of outpatients felt unable to comment because they had met too few of the particular people we were asking about.

Table 10.6 shows that 80% of outpatients of all ages, (including the parents of child patients) felt that all the nurses they had met at the hospital were considerate to them, 88% thought all the para-medical staff—physiotherapists, dieticians, radiographers, technicians and so on, had been nice to them, and 84% had found all the non-medical staff helpful—porters, receptionists, orderlies etc. Less than 5% of patients found on their visits to hospital that the majority of the staff they met (nurses, para-medical staff, and non-medical staff) were either inconsiderate, unhelpful or in some way not nice to them.

Table 10.6   Proportions of outpatients who were satisfied with the attitude of various groups of hospital staff they met on their visits to hospital

Proportions of staff who were considerate, nice, or helpful	Attitude of hospital staff		
	nursing staff who were considerate	para-medical staff who were nice to patients[1]	non-medical staff who were helpful
	%	%	%
all	80	88	84
most	17	10	12
only a few	3	2	4
Base=100%[2]	2114	1673	1765

1. physiotherapists, radiographers, dieticians etc.
2. base=all outpatients who met sufficient staff to be able to comment

35. Of the 49 patients who minded not being asked, 22 also objected to the students being present.

It may be of interest to note that if the views of outpatients are compared with those of inpatients, significantly higher proportions of outpatients regarded *all* the nurses as considerate and *all* the non-medical staff as being helpful. Whereas 80% of outpatients found all the nurses considerate, and 84% thought all the non-medical staff were helpful, the corresponding proportions for the inpatient sample were 64% and 80% respectively. However very similar, and only small proportions of both outpatients and inpatients felt that only a few of the nurses were considerate and only a few of the non-medical staff helpful.

11.0 Discharge from hospital and after care
Inpatients only

The care a hospital provides for a patient does not end at the time of discharge; arrangements for getting the patient home and for helping them manage once they are there, follow-up checks or treatment as an outpatient, and liaison with the patient's own family doctor, are all aspects of after care in which the hospital plays an important part. If they are mismanaged or inadequate, they may leave patients with an unfavourable impression of the hospital, even though they may have otherwise been satisfied with the treatment they received and the conditions and facilities in the hospital.

11.1 Arrangements for getting home from hospital

In the same way as a few patients felt they originally had been given too little notice of admission, so a number of patients felt they were not given enough warning of their discharge. The data show that 12% of all inpatients felt there was insufficient time once they were told they could go home to make any arrangements that were necessary. There was some evidence that elderly patients were less likely to have worried about this than younger patients; only 6% of patients aged 65 and over felt they were given too little notice that they were being discharged compared with 14% of patients under 65.

One in ten inpatients was taken home from hospital by ambulance or by hospital car, and of the 716 patients who made their own arrangements for getting home 60 (8%) would have preferred hospital transport to have been laid on. This includes four patients who although they would have found an ambulance more comfortable and convenient, nevertheless decided to make their own way home rather than wait, possibly several hours, until an ambulance was available.

A significantly greater proportion of patients aged 65 and over were taken home by ambulance (31%) compared to those under 65 (5%); however elderly patients who had made their own arrangements for getting home were no more likely than younger patients to have said they would have preferred hospital transport to have been laid on.

Just over half the patients who would have preferred hospital transport to have been laid on, were worried about the effect of a journey on their medical condition, while the remainder would have preferred hospital transport for other, non-medical reasons. The most frequently mentioned of such reasons was that someone, usually a relative, had to come to collect them, and this often meant their taking time off work. Seven patients mentioned the expense of taking a taxi, and a small number of patients were mainly concerned about the inconvenience of waiting for and using public transport.

11.2 Worries about leaving hospital

The majority of patients (86%) were quite happy to leave hospital when they did, but 5% felt they should have been discharged earlier and 9% that they should have stayed in hospital longer. As can be seen from table 11.1 below, quite a high proportion of maternity patients (16%) felt they could have gone home sooner but an analysis by age showed that almost all the elderly patients spoken to (93%) were satisfied that they had been discharged at about the right time.

Table 11.1   Proportions of men and women patients who felt they should have stayed longer in hospital

Patients opinion of time of discharge	Men	Women		Men and women
		maternity patients	non-maternity patients	
	%	%	%	%
should have stayed in longer	9	7	10	9
should have been discharged sooner	4	16	3	5
discharged at about the right time	87	77	87	86
Base: all inpatients=100%	307	97	393	797

Worries about managing at home

Although most patients were quite happy to leave hospital when they did about one in six patients had some worries or doubts about how they would manage once they were home. Obviously patients who felt they should have been kept in hospital longer were more likely to have worries about managing at home than those who were happy to be discharged when they were, but analysis showed that many mothers of new babies, some 16% of whom it has already been seen felt they should have been discharged sooner, were nevertheless worried about coping at home: nearly one in three had doubts of this sort. As can be seen from the table below, other women patients, probably because of their greater domestic responsibilities were also more likely than men to have doubts about how they would manage.

Table 11.2   Proportions of men and women patients who were worried about being able to manage at home

Whether worried about ability to manage at home	Men	Women		Men and women
		maternity patients	non-maternity patients	
	%	%	%	%
Yes worried	15	30	18	18
No, not worried	85	70	82	82
Base: all inpatients= 100%[1]	307	97	393	797

1. includes the parents of child patients who answered in terms of whether they were worried about coping with the child at home

An analysis by age showed no differences other than those which could be explained by differences in the sex composition of the groups or by the presence of maternity patients, with the exception that only 6% of men aged 65 and over were found to have worries of this sort, a significantly smaller proportion compared to that for either younger men or women of the same age. It may be that elderly men and particularly those living alone have fewer worries about coping because help has been arranged for them, by, for example, the social services department, but further analysis showed that just over one in four of all inpatients living alone had doubts about their ability to manage once they had left hospital.

The hospital social worker

One in six inpatients (including the parents of child patients) were visited by a hospital social worker soon after they were admitted to hospital; of the 656 patients (and parents) who did not see the social worker 5% had general worries or problems at that stage, about for example, their job, their family, or financial matters that they would have liked to have been able to talk over with the social worker. Just under one in four of the 144 patients who, while they were still in hospital, had worries about how they would manage at home once they had been discharged, talked to a social worker about their doubts, but nearly half of those who had not seen the social worker would have liked to have seen someone with whom they could discuss these problems.

Thus it can be calculated that 4% of all inpatients would have liked the opportunity to talk to the hospital social worker soon after they were admitted, and 6% of all inpatients would have liked to talk to the social worker before they were discharged about the doubts they had concerning their ability to manage at home.

For 21 of the 34 patients who talked to a social worker about the problems they might have once they were home, help was arranged; home helps, meals-on-wheels, and providing special aids for self-care were the most frequent areas where help was provided. One lady was put in touch by the hospital social worker with an organisation formed to help people with multiple sclerosis, and two patients were told how to go about getting some financial assistance to help them while they were away from work.

Managing at home

Despite the fact that 18% of inpatients initially had worries about how they would cope at home, and 9% felt they should have been kept in hospital for a longer period, 95% of all inpatients said that once they got home they managed all right (this again includes parents of child patients). Generally patients were satisfied that they had been given enough help and advice by the hospital about managing at home; 94% of all inpatients said the hospital had done all they could to help them. Twenty two of the 45 patients who felt the hospital could have done more would have liked the hospital to have arranged for domiciliary visits by a district nurse or health visitor: they said they felt that the hospital should check that patients were following the advice they had been given, but one suspects that these patients wanted the reassurance of someone 'keeping an eye on them'. Sixteen patients felt the hospital should have arranged domestic help for them at home.

Small numbers of patients would have liked more information from the hospital, either about how long they should stay off work, (or how long their children should be away from school) or as to how they should expect their condition to progress—what to regard as normal after an operation or spell in hospital, and a few mothers felt they could have been better prepared for the amount of work that a new baby involved.

11.3 Communication between the hospital and the patient's GP

It may not only be important from the medical point of view that a patient's GP is aware of the outcome of their stay in hospital, but it may also be disconcerting for the patient to feel that his family doctor is unaware of what has been happening.

Of the 797 inpatients in the sample, 139 had not seen their family doctor between being discharged from hospital and being interviewed, however 15 (11%) of these 139 patients had been given a letter by the hospital to give to their doctor when they saw him.

A further 64 patients had seen their doctor since being discharged but could not remember how soon after their discharge it had been; as nearly half these patients were also not sure whether or not their doctor had heard from the hospital they have been excluded both from table 11.3 below and from the discussion that follows. Additionally, 76 patients, although they could remember when it was they first saw their GP, did not have a letter to give their GP and were not certain whether he had heard from the hospital about the outcome of their stay; these 76 patients are also excluded from the table.

Of the remaining inpatients who could remember their first visit to, or by, their GP since their discharge from hospital, just over half (58%) said their doctor had already heard from the hospital, and a further 19% had a letter from the hospital to their doctor which they took with them on their first visit. However, there remained 23% who were certain their doctor had not heard from the hospital about how they had got on, and who did not have a letter from the hospital to give to their doctor. It can be seen from table 11.3 that the interval between being discharged and first seeing a GP had only a marginal effect on the likelihood of the doctor being informed, either direct from the hospital or by letter brought by the patient, of the outcome of their patient's stay in hospital. Not surprisingly however, doctors who saw their patients within three days of their discharge were less likely by that time to have heard direct from the hospital, than those whose patients waited longer before seeing them.

Table 11.3 Proportions of inpatients who, on their first visit to their GP after discharge, found their doctor did not know about the outcome of their stay in hospital

How GP had heard about outcome of patient's stay in hospital	Interval between discharge from hospital and first seeing GP				
	less than 3 days	3 days—less than 1 week	1 week—less than 2 weeks	2 weeks—less than 1 month	1 month or more
	%	%	%	%	%
Patient did not have a letter and was sure GP had not heard from hospital	25	21	30	19	15
GP had heard from hospital	48	61	59	60	75
Patient had letter to give GP	27	18	11	21	10
Base=100%[1]	181	109	83	53	84

1. Base=all inpatients excluding those who had not yet seen their GP, those who could not remember when they first saw him after their discharge, and those who had no letter from the hospital and were not certain whether he had heard from the hospital.

12.0   A note on parent's attitudes to their child's stay in hospital

Of the 797 patients interviewed on the inpatient study, 97 were children aged under 14.

Of these 97 children almost all (95%) had stayed in a children's or babies ward, the remaining five children were in wards with adults. Only one of the parents of the five children who were in wards with adults would have preferred their child to have been in a children's ward, and 86% of those whose children were in children's wards were happy with this arrangement. The preference for a children's ward was not related to the age of the child, and the main reason given by parents in support of this preference was the company that the child would have being with other children.

Eight out of ten parents were satisfied with the facilities and condition of the ward their child was in; the complaints from the few parents who were dissatisfied were various and included there being too few toys or play facilities, too few washing and toilet facilities, the ward being underheated or in need of decoration, and complaints about children being put into cots when they were used to sleeping in a bed at home.

Only 12% of mothers had been asked if they would like to stay in hospital with their child overnight or longer, and half of those who were asked did in fact stay. All but one felt the arrangements were satisfactory; the only complaint was from a mother who had to leave her child when she went for a meal—she would have preferred to have stayed with her child and had meals brought to her. Of the 77 mothers who were not asked if they wanted to stay, 18 (23%) would have liked to have done so; the rest did not feel it was necessary.

Eight out of ten parents said the hospital was happy for them to phone up at any time to find out how their child was, only four parents got the impression the hospital did not really like it, and the remainder had not found it necessary to phone at odd times and so could not say. The vast majority of parents (90 out of 97) were in favour of hospitals encouraging parents to spend some time at the hospital helping and keeping the children amused.

13.0 A note on dissatisfaction with the service

It would be unrealistic to expect every user of any service to be completely satisfied, and this study has shown that there were varying proportions of patients dissatisfied with most of the examined aspects of both the inpatient and outpatient service.

It has not yet been shown whether most patients have a few complaints, or whether a few patients have many complaints.

13.1 Inpatients

The table below shows various aspects of the service with which more than 10% of patients were dissatisfied.

Table 13.1   Aspects of hospital service with which more than 10% of inpatients were dissatisfied

Aspect of service	% dissatisfied
Based on part sample:[1]	
emergencies: waiting for attention	26
non-emergencies: waiting for admission	20
objected to smoking in ward/hospital room	16
Based on total adult sample (aged 14 and over)[1]	
woken too early	43
food	21
washing and bathing facilities	19
toilet facilities	15
comfort of beds	13
noise during daytime	12
privacy during examination and treatment	11
Based on total sample (all ages)[1]	
information about progress	31
difficulty understanding doctors (apart from using medical terms)	15
notice of discharge	12

1. excluding 'no answers'

Where only a small proportion of the total inpatient sample was dissatisfied with a particular aspect of the service, either because it did not affect them or because they did not use the facility, it could be argued that any improvement would make little difference to the overall number of inpatients who would have no complaints. For example, 26% of emergency admissions who had to wait to see a doctor on arrival at hospital felt that their wait was unreasonable, but this represents only 7% of emergencies, and only 3% of the total inpatient sample.

For the purpose of this analysis, five aspects of the service were examined, of

which, all, or at least all adult inpatients, would have had experience . . .
>   waking times
>   privacy during examination and treatment
>   information about progress
>   understanding doctors (apart from their use of medical terminology)
> and notice of discharge;

plus a further two aspects which together covered the whole sample . . .
>   emergencies—waiting for attention
> and non emergencies—waiting for admission.

This made six aspects in all.

By looking at all combinations of dissatisfaction with these six aspects of the service, it was found that 36% of all inpatients were satisfied with all six aspects, and a further 30% were dissatisfied with only one aspect; 29% had two or three causes of dissatisfaction, 5% had four or five, but no-one was dissatisfied with all six aspects.

If those dissatisfied with only one of these six aspects were all complaining about the same thing, then clearly by improving that aspect of the service, the proportion of patients with no complaints about any of the aspects investigated would rise from 36% to 66%. However this was not so; of the inpatients with only one source of dissatisfaction . . .
>   56% complained of being woken too early
>   21% said they were not told enough about how they were progressing
>   7% had difficulty in understanding what the doctors were saying
>   7% were not given enough notice of discharge
>   8% were either dissatisfied with how long they had to wait for attention,
>   or for a hospital bed to become available
> and for 1% their sole source of dissatisfaction was the lack of privacy during
>   examination or treatment.

However, the two main sources of complaint for those dissatisfied with only one aspect of the service, waking times and lack of communication, also together accounted for over a third of all patients dissatisfied with *two* aspects of the service.

If therefore ward routine could be changed to avoid waking patients until after 7.00 am, then the proportion of inpatients satisfied with all six aspects would rise from 36% to around 54%; even if patients were not woken until after 6.30 am then at least 50% would have no complaints about any of the aspects examined (table 6.3 refers).

If improvements could be made in communications, by telling the patient more about their treatment and progress, *as well as changing waking times,* then two thirds of the inpatients would have no complaints (about any of the aspects examined).

It is worth noting that while some 30% of those under 65 years old were satisfied with all six aspects of the service, the corresponding proportion for those aged at least 65 was nearly twice as great: 57%. Where the elderly did complain, it was usually about one aspect only, waking time causing most dissatisfaction, followed by wanting to know more about their treatment and progress.

13.2 Outpatients

A similar analysis of dissatisfaction was carried out on the outpatient sample and produced the following results:

Table 13.2 Aspects of the hospital service with which more than 10% of outpatients were dissatisfied

Aspect of service	% dissatisfied
Based on part sample:[1]	
no toys for children in waiting room (child patients only)	47
getting a satisfactory answer from the doctor to questions about progress	37
time spent waiting for hospital transport home	28
ambulance making a detour to collect other patients and take them to hospital	23
waiting for a first appointment	21
Based on total sample (all ages)[1]	
information about progress	25
length of time spent at the hospital	19
adequacy of space in waiting room	18
length of wait before seeing doctor	16
difficulty understanding medical terminology	15
other difficulty in understanding doctor	15
appearance of waiting room	14
number of seats in waiting room	11

1. excluding 'no answers'

As was found for the inpatient sample, in most cases only a relatively small proportion of outpatients were dissatisfied with any particular aspect of the service, and there were many aspects not listed above which caused dissatisfaction to 10% or less of the sample.

The six factors used in the outpatient analysis were as follows:
information about progress
length of time spent at the hospital
adequacy of space in waiting room
appearance of waiting room
length of wait before seeing doctor
understanding doctors (other than use of medical terminology)

Inspection of the levels of dissatisfaction with all combinations of these six factors showed that 46% of outpatients were satisfied with all six aspects and 24% were dissatisfied with one only; 24% had two or three complaints, 6% had four or five, and no-one was dissatisfied with all six aspects of the service.

Of the outpatients with one complaint only:

37% wanted more information about their progress
17% complained that the waiting room was overcrowded
15% found the waiting room drab and depressing
14% had trouble understanding what the doctors were saying
11% felt that they spent too long at the hospital
and 6% thought that they had an unreasonable wait before seeing the
doctor.

It can be seen that the most frequent complaint from outpatients dissatisfied with only one aspect of the service, was that they were given insufficient information about their progress and treatment; if this could be remedied the proportion of outpatients satisfied with all six aspects would increase from 46% to 56%.

If the two most frequent single causes of dissatisfaction, lack of information and overcrowding of the waiting room, could both be alleviated only a further 4% of patients would be satisfied with all six aspects making 60% in all.

As with the inpatient sample a much higher proportion of elderly patients were satisfied with all six aspects of the hospital service: 63% of those aged 65 and over had no complaints compared with 42% of those aged under 65. Again, most elderly patients who were dissatisfied had only one complaint, and this was, most frequently, that they wanted more information about their progress. A somewhat smaller proportion had difficulty only in understanding what the doctors were saying.

Appendix I

Details of the sample design and selection[36]

by Elizabeth Breeze

The survey covering the United Kingdom, collected data from both people who had been outpatients and from people who had been inpatients. Outpatients were defined as those who had attended a hospital casualty or outpatient department (excluding routine pre- or post natal visits) during a specified period. Inpatients were those who had been in hospital overnight or longer during a specified period. Ideally the hospital experiences would be recent to avoid changes in hospital practice confounding the results and, of course, to avoid recall problems for the patient.

From General Household Survey data it is known that approximately 10% of persons of all ages are outpatients during a three month period, and that under 2% are inpatients. It was therefore considered too expensive to take a random sample of the general population and sift out all those with no hospital experience.

The samples in Great Britain

Independent samples of outpatients and inpatients were taken partly to avoid confusion between the two types of experience in the patient's mind, and partly for practical reasons as part of the sample design.

The outpatient sample

The sample was derived from respondents to the 1976 General Household Survey (GHS). This survey is a multi-purpose continuing survey in which members of over 10,000 households are interviewed annually. Subject areas covered by the survey include housing, employment and health. The 1976 GHS schedule included the question . . .

"during the three months prior to interview did you attend as a patient the casualty or outpatient department of a hospital (apart from straightforward ante or post natal visits)?"

Anyone answering yes to this question was eligible for the survey. The sample thereby produced is of individuals who have been outpatients during a 3 month period between October 1975 and November 1976 inclusive. The GHS sample design ensures a widespread coverage of the general population; electoral wards are stratified by region, a socio-economic group indicator and by an owner-occupation factor, and one ward is selected per quarter from each of the 168 strata so formed, hence our sample was spread over 672 wards. Although this makes fieldwork less economical than one would wish it does increase the likelihood of representing all types of experience by increasing the number of hospitals attended.

---

36. Papers giving more detail of the sample design, outlining the problems involved in using a recall sample and validating the sample, are in preparation and will be available from Social Survey Division.

IDENTIFICATION OF SAMPLE

The sample of outpatients was obtained by a computer sift of all individual data-sets from the 1976 GHS.

At every household cooperating on the GHS one member (usually head of household or housewife) is asked if they would agree to a recall interview should any government department require further information. The name of this person is recorded and was also given to interviewers. Any household which had refused permission to recall was not approached.

SAMPLE SIZE

The time and resource constraints on the survey precluded detailed analysis of subgroups of the population. However, the variety of experience possible warranted a sample of the order of 2,500. From previous years' results it was anticipated that there would be roughly 3,000 outpatients in a year's GHS sample. It was decided that all eligible outpatients should be included to yield an estimated achieved sample of 2,600 interviews.

Inpatient sample

A random sample of the general population, sifting out all those with no inpatient experience was rejected as both too expensive and time-consuming. The use of hospital records to provide a sample of inpatients was also rejected since there was insufficient opportunity to obtain clearance for using this source, and then to make suitable arrangements for obtaining the sample.

There is no suitable standard question on the GHS asking about inpatient experiences. However it was suggested that additional questions be added to the GHS schedule using a trailer system.

SAMPLE SIZE

Sample size was again constrained by the time that would be available for analysis, and also by the number of eligible individuals that could be identified by the GHS. It was estimated that a minimum of 800 achieved interviews would be required, and if the trailer question on the GHS schedule covered a 12 month reference period and was asked over two quarters, it was estimated that something of the order of 1,000 eligible individuals might be identified.

TRAILER SYSTEM

The trailer consisted of an extra sheet tagged onto the main GHS schedules. Interviewers recorded details of any inpatient spells during the reference period, together with the sex and age of the individuals concerned (to give a basic demographic profile of the eligible population). They then asked the inpatients if they would be willing to cooperate at a further interview specifically about their inpatient experiences. The trailer sheets were self-contained so could be detached from the main schedules and processed in advance of other GHS data. In this way a list of eligible individuals was obtained within weeks of the GHS interviews whereas data cannot be extracted from the main schedules until several months after the interview. As in the outpatient sample people who had refused a recall interview were not approached.

Although both inpatient and outpatient samples were derived from GHS in Great Britain it should be stressed that they were independent samples and it would be incorrect to combine the results.

Northern Ireland

As the General Household Survey does not extend to Northern Ireland separate arrangements had to be made. Samples of outpatients and inpatients could only be obtained via a sift process ie a general sample of addresses taken and eligible individuals at those addresses identified. This was feasible in Northern Ireland because only a small sample was required and the Survey Unit in Northern Ireland had the resources available.

To give households and hence eligible individuals the same chance of selection in Northern Ireland as Great Britain the initial samples of households should be in the same proportion to the GHS samples as the total number of households in each part of the UK. The ratio of households in Northern Ireland to households in Great Britain was calculated from 1971 Census data and applied to the initial GHS sample size. This yielded a set sample size of 341 addresses. Instead of taking an independent sample half this size for inpatients it was decided to derive both samples from the same set of 341 addresses, include all eligible outpatients and subsample one in two of the inpatients to restore the correct probability. Addresses of domestic rateable units were sampled from the Valuation List.

A postal form was sent to each address and reminders were sent to addresses from which there had been no response at two and again at four weeks after the initial mailing. From the returns addresses containing no eligible individuals were excluded. Interviewers visited the remaining addresses and having checked that the named persons ticked as outpatient/inpatient were eligible, interviewed them. An individual was eligible as an outpatient if he had attended an outpatient or casualty department between 1st May 1977 and 31st July 1977, or as an inpatient if he had been in hospital between 1st August 1976 and 31st July 1977. These periods make the Northern Ireland samples comparable to the Great Britain samples with respect to length of reference period. It should be noted that the outpatient dates were more recent in Northern Ireland. This is not ideal since there could have been changes in practice between 1976 and 1977; however the numbers involved are so small that bias should be negligible.

Interdependence of samples

Unlike the samples in Great Britain the samples of outpatients and inpatients were not independent in Northern Ireland. An individual could be selected both as outpatient and inpatient but it was thought unreasonable to interview anyone with respect to both experiences so the following procedure was adopted: the individual concerned was given a full inpatient interview and some basic data on number of outpatient visits collected. These persons are then effectively losses from the outpatient sample; although they are not a random subsample their numbers are negligible compared to total UK sample size.

Response rates and non-response from original GHS respondents: *outpatient and inpatient samples in Great Britain*

	Outpatient sample		Inpatient sample	
	Nos	%	Nos	%
Outpatients identified on GHS:	3058 =	100.00	962 =	100.00
excluded: did not agree to recall	187 ⎫		⎫	
already been recalled on	112[1] ⎬ =	12.50	⎬ 51 =	5.30
other	85 ⎭		⎭	
Sample issued for interview	2674 =	100.00	911 =	100.00
ineligible: died	66 ⎫		⎫	
denied hospital experience	48 ⎬ =	4.41	⎬ 37 =	4.06
other	4 ⎭		⎭	
Total eligible sample:	2556 =	100.00	874 =	100.00
non-contacts	193 =	7.55	45	5.15
refusals: anti surveys	37 ⎫		⎫	
too ill/confused	18 ⎬ =	3.95	⎬ 38 =	4.35
other	46 ⎭		⎭	
Achieved interviews:	2262 =	88.49	791 =	90.50
withdrawn: private patient	19 ⎫ =	1.53	22 ⎫ =	2.63
other reasons[2]	20 ⎭		1 ⎭	
Total interviews for analysis	2223	86.97	768	87.87

1. already visited for another follow-up survey of GHS respondents
2. inadequate information or found to be ineligible—visit outside reference period, not visited a hospital etc

Response rates and non-response to postal questionnaire and at interview stages: *outpatient and inpatient samples in Northern Ireland*

	Nos	%
Original addresses issued:	341 =	100
non response	60	17

	Outpatient sample		Inpatient sample	
	Nos	%	Nos	%
Patients identified by postal:	104 =	100	83 =	100
withdrawn had both outpatient and				
inpatient experience	28	27	—[1]	
Sample issued for interview:	76 =	100	83 =	100
ineligible[2]	31	41	20	24
Total eligible sample	45 =	100	63 =	100
non-contacts	—		4	
refusals	1		—	
Achieved interviews	44	98	59	94
Total interviews for analysis	44		29	
			(1 in 2 subsample)	

1. the 28 patients who had both inpatient and outpatient experience were *excluded* from the outpatient sample, but remained as part of the inpatient sample
2. mainly cases where the experience was not within the reference period

Appendix II

The trailer questions used on the General Household Survey to identify people with outpatient and inpatient experience living in private households in England and Wales.

The postal questionnaire used to identify people with outpatient and inpatient experience living in Northern Ireland.

The covering letter and reminder letters sent with the postal questionnaire in Northern Ireland.

The outpatient questionnaire (GB)

The inpatient questionnaire (GB)

S457/1977/1
Quarters 2 and 3

To be checked for all households coded 10 or 21-24 on Interview Record

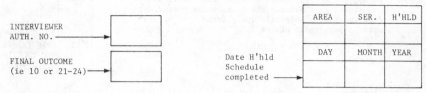

INTERVIEWER
AUTH. NO. ———————▶

FINAL OUTCOME
(ie 10 or 21-24)———▶

Date H'hld
Schedule
completed ———▶

	AREA	SER.	H'HLD
	DAY	MONTH	YEAR

CHECK FOR EVERY MEMBER OF THE HOUSEHOLD, <u>INCLUDING CHILDREN</u>

INTRODUCE

1. During the 12 months ending yesterday has anyone in
   this household been in hospital as an inpatient
   overnight or longer?
   (REMEMBER Q.11 OF HEALTH SECTION)

   IF YES ——▶ASK Qs.2-5
   IF NO ——▶DO NOT COMPLETE
            THIS SHEET

FOR EACH INPATIENT

ENTER PERSON NO.
OF INPATIENT AND ▶
IF PROXY RING 9

2. How many times? (WRITE IN) ——————▶

FOR EACH VISIT

3. What month and year did you leave hospital?

	1st spell	2nd spell	3rd spell	1st spell	2nd spell	3rd spell
(person no.)			9			9
Currently in hospital	1	1	1	1	1	1
Month (WRITE IN NO.) ———▶ January = 01, February = 02 etc						
Year (RING): 1976	6	6	6	6	6	6
1977	7	7	7	7	7	7

4. Was this as a medical, surgical
   (or maternity) patient?

	1st spell	2nd spell	3rd spell	1st spell	2nd spell	3rd spell
Medical/surgical	1	1	1	1	1	1
Maternity	2	2	2	2	2	2
Other	3	3	3	3	3	3

5. We may be doing a survey for the Royal
   Commission on the NHS at the end of
   the year. If we do, please could   Yes ..
   we come and talk to you again?   No ...

Yes	1	1
No	2	2

IF YES: ENTER NAME OF   Mr/Mrs/Miss ———▶
        INPATIENT

                         First name ———▶

              and   Surname ———▶

INTERVIEWER

Transfer this information   Age (WRITE IN)—▶
for each inpatient, whether
permission given to recall   Sex: Male ....
or not   Female .....

Male	1	1
Female	2	2

The trailer question used on the General Household Survey
to identify people with outpatient experience

TO ALL

6. During the months of ....., ... and ....., did
   you attend as a patient the casualty or outpatient
   department of a hospital (apart from straightforward
   ante or post-natal visits)?

	CODE	
Yes	1	ASK (a)-(b)
No	2	GO TO Q.10
		PAGE 40

IF YES

(a) Which month was this?

(b) How many times did you attend in that month?

		EARLIEST MONTH IN REFERENCE PERIOD	CODE	SECOND MONTH IN REFERENCE PERIOD	CODE	THIRD MONTH IN REFERENCE PERIOD	CODE
(a)	Month ——→						
(b)	No.of times	——————→	.....	——————→	......	——————→	......

		CODE 1st SEQ.	CODE 2nd SEQ.	CODE 3rd SEQ.	CODE 4th SEQ.
(f)	Which clinic or department of outpatients did you attend?				
	PRIORITY CODE → Casualty/accident/emergency ...	2	2	2	2
	CODE — Physiotherapy	3	3	3	3
	ALL — X-ray (DEEP X-RAY OR RADIUM				
	THAT — TREATMENT = CODE 5).....	4	4	4	4
	APPLY — Other (SPECIFY)...............	5	5	5	5

SEQUENCE NO. ....

SEQUENCE NO. ....

SEQUENCE NO. ....

SEQUENCE NO. ....

136

The postal questionnaire used to identify people with outpatient and inpatient experience living in Northern Ireland

---

	Your reference
	Our reference
	Date

HOW TO COMPLETE THIS FORM:

1. START: by listing below everyone living at the address printed on the label above, giving each persons full name, age, and sex. (There is more room on the back of this form if you need it).

2. THEN: in the column headed 'INPATIENTS' put a tick (✓) against the name of anyone who has been to hospital as an INPATIENT at anytime since AUGUST 1st 1976.

3. FINALLY: in the column headed 'OUTPATIENTS' put a tick against the name of anyone who has been to hospital as an OUTPATIENT or CASUALTY at anytime since MAY 1st 1977.

Surname (IN BLOCK CAPITALS PLEASE)	First name	Age last birthday	Tick which applies Male	Female	INPATIENTS	OUTPATIENTS
1.						
2.						
3.						
4.						
5.						
6.						
7.						
8.						
9.						

NOW PLEASE RETURN THIS FORM IN THE ENVELOPE PROVIDED - EVEN IF NO-ONE HAS BEEN TO HOSPITAL SO THAT WE DO NOT HAVE TO TROUBLE YOU FURTHER FOR IT. THANK YOU FOR HELPING US.

The covering letter sent with the postal questionnaire in
Northern Ireland

Dear

As you may know a Royal Commission has been set up to look at the workings of the National Health Service and to see whether any changes should be made which would improve the service. Part of the Commission's job has been to listen to the views of individuals and bodies concerned with, or working in the Health Service, and we are co-operating in a survey to be carried out in Great Britain to find out from the general public their experiences and opinion of the National Health Service.

We are particularly interested in knowing what use is being made of the hospital service, and would be very grateful if you could complete the attached sheet showing who lives at the address printed on the label and whether anybody has been to hospital either as an outpatient or casualty at anytime since May 1st 1977, or as an inpatient since August 1st 1976. Please include anyone who lives at the address on the label even if they belong to a different family or household and also include anyone who is temporarily away from home eg. on holiday, at school, in hospital. Any information you give will be treated in strict confidence.

Later in the year our interviewers will be calling at some of the addresses we are writing to inviting people to tell us about their experiences, but it is very important that all households complete the form since only by getting a representative sample of households can we hope to give the Royal Commission evidence on which they could suggest improvements to the Health Service for the future.

I should therefore be most grateful if you could complete the enclosed form and return it to me in the envelope provided: no stamp is required.

Thank you very much for your help and co-operation.

Yours sincerely

1st Reminder

On   I sent you a letter asking for your help in a survey we are planning to carry out to find out peoples' experiences and opinions of the National Health Service.

Up to the present we have not had a reply from you and I would be grateful if you could let me have the completed form back as soon as possible, showing who lives at this address, even if there is no-one there who has had any personal experience of the hospital service.

If you have already returned the form within the last few days, please disregard this letter.

Thank you for your help and co-operation.

2nd Reminder

On   I sent you a letter asking for your help in a survey we are planning to carry out to find out peoples' experiences and opinions of the National Health Service.

In order to get an unbiased picture it is necessary that everyone be given an equal chance of being asked their opinions. I would therefore be grateful if you could complete the form and return it as soon as possible, showing who lives at this address and whether anybody has been to hospital either as an outpatient or casualty since May 1st 1977 or as an inpatient since August 1st 1976. I enclose another form and a copy of my letter in case the originals have gone astray.

If you have already replied within the last few days, please disregard this letter.

Thank you for your help and co-operation.

Serial number

(i) Interviewers name _____

(ii) Authorisation number _____

(iii) Date of interview   /   /197

(iv) Interview with: sampled person aged 14 or over.......   1

                 proxy taken for sampled person under
                   14 years   2

                 relationship of proxy (specify)

Copy from sampling sheet before interview:

(a) Date of GHS interview   /197

                              month   year

(b) Outpatient details:

Sex		Age	Marital Status		
M	F		M	S	W/D
1	2		1	2	3

(c) Outpatient visits:

	Reference period	No. of visits	
Month:	_____	None 0	Other specify
Month:	_____	None 0	Other specify
Month:	_____	None 0	Other specify
		Total no. of visits	=

(d) Departments visited during 3 - month reference period:

                  Consultative outpatients   1

CODE ALL   Casualty/accident/emergency   2

THAT APPLY   Other ancillary (physio. X-ray)   3

                  Other   4

1. Before I ask you anything about your visit(s) to the hospital as an outpatient, from your own experience would you personally say that on the whole the hospital service for outpatients is ...

RUNNING PROMPT	very good	1
	good	2
	has its faults	3
	or is poor?	4

IF <u>MORE THAN ONE VISIT</u> IN THREE MONTH REFERENCE PERIOD GO ONTO Q13 PAGE 6

Qs 2 - 12 APPLY <u>TO ALL WITH ONLY ONE VISIT</u> IN THREE MONTH REFERENCE PERIOD

2. When you went to hospital as an outpatient in _____ 197__, what was it for?

[Give full details of condition, symptoms, treatment]

CONDITION

A

3. What was the name of the hospital you went to on that occasion?

specify: _____

4. And when you went were you seen as a National Health Service patient or as a private patient?

National Health Service .	1
Private patient	2

5. Did you have an appointment to go along to the
   hospital on that day, or did you go straight to
   the hospital without an appointment?

Had an appointment	1	
No appointment	2	onto Q11

6. Was this the first time you had been to ... hosp ...
   as an outpatient about your ....., or had you
   been to the same hospital as an outpatient before
   about it?

First time	1	onto Q8
Had been before	2	

7. So when was the first time you went to ... hosp ...
   as an outpatient, about your .....?

before 1975	1	onto Q10
1975	2	
1976	3	

8. How long did you have to wait for this first
   appointment at ... hosp ...?

1 week or less (7 days or less) ......:	1	onto Q10
Over 1 week up to 2 weeks (8 - 14 days)	2	
Over 2 weeks up to 3 weeks (15 - 21 days)	3	
Over 3 weeks up to 4 weeks (21 - 28 days)	4	ask Q9
Over 4 weeks up to 5 weeks	5	
Over 5 weeks up to 6 weeks	6	
Over 6 weeks (specify no. of weeks) _____	7	

9. Did you mind waiting that long for the appointment
   or didn't it really matter that much?

Minded waiting	1	ask (a)
Didn't really matter	2	

IF MINDED WAITING (1)

(a) Why did you mind having to wait for an
    appointment?

    0

TO ALL

10. Who first referred you to ... hosp ... about your
    .....?

GP, family doctor ....:..........	1
Private consultant or specialist ...	2
O/P dept. at another hospital	3
Referred after spell as in-patient .	4
Casualty, accident, emergency	5
Other (specify)	6

142

11. Apart from the visit you made in ... ref. month ...
    197 have you had to go to ... hosp ... since then
    about your .....?

Yes, had to go again	1	ask (a)
No, that was last/only visit ...	2	onto Q26 page 14

IF YES HAD TO GO AGAIN (1)

(a) Are you still going to ..... about your .....
    or have you finished going now?

Still going	1
Finished going	2

12. So when was your last appointment at ... hosp ...
    for your .....?

    specify: □□ / 1 9 7 □
              month   year

onto Q26 p.14

[NOW GO ONTO Q26 PAGE 14]

Qs 13 - 25 APPLY TO ALL WITH MORE THAN ONE VISIT IN
THREE MONTH PERIOD

INTERVIEWER TO COPY FROM FRONT PAGE OF QUESTIONNAIRE

Total no. of visits in 3 - month reference period→ ☐

---

13. I'd like to talk first of all about your visits
to hospital as an outpatient between ..... and
..... 197 .

[START WITH FIRST VISIT IN EARLIEST OF 3 MONTHS]

If we start with the first visit you made in 197
what did you go to hospital for on that occasion?

[Give full details of
conditions, symptoms,
treatment]

CONDITION

A

---

14. I believe you went to hospital as an outpatient
..... times between ... and 197   , how many
of these visits were for your ... cond. A ...?

All visits in period for cond. A   x   onto Q17

Only some visits for cond.A. Specify number→ ☐

144

TO ALL WITH VISITS FOR MORE THAN ONE CONDITION

15. So what were the other visits you made
    to hospital at that time for?

    [Give full details of
      condition, symptoms,
      treatment]

         CONDITION

    # B

         CONDITION

    # C

16. And how many times did you go to hospital
    as an outpatient between ... and 197   , about
    .....

         condition B?   specify no. of visits ⟶ ☐

         condition C?   specify no. of visits ⟶ ☐

    INTERVIEWER TO CODE AND CHECK:

                   Total no. of visits
                   for conditions A + B + C ⟶ ☐

    [CHECK THAT THIS TOTAL AGREES WITH TOTAL
      IN BOX AT TOP OF PAGE 6..

      IF AFTER CHECKING, TOTALS DISAGREE, TAKE
      INFORMANTS ESTIMATE AND MAKE FULL NOTES.]

ASK Qs 17 - 25 ABOUT CONDITION A AND CODE/WRITE ANSWERS IN COL A ─────────────
[IF MADE VISITS FOR MORE THAN ONE CONDITION, REPEAT Qs 17 - 25 FOR EACH CONDITION
IN TURN : CODE/WRITE ANSWERS IN APPROPRIATE COLUMN]────────────────────

Interviewer: First specify no. of visits made──▶

17. Introduce: You said you made ..... visits to hospital between ... and
..... 197 about your ...... Thinking now about the first of these
visits you made during that period ...
What was the name of the hospital you went to on that
occasion?

Specify:

18. When you went were you seen as a National Health Service patient
or as a private patient?

National Health Service ....

Private patient ....

19. Did you have an appointment to go along to the hospital on that
day, or did you go straight to the hospital without an
appointment?

Had an appointment ....

No appointment ....

20. Was this the first time you had been to ... hosp. ... as an
outpatient about your ...., or had you been to the same hospital
before as an outpatient about it?

First time ....

Had been before ....

CONDITION A	CONDITION B	CONDITION C
No. of visits ☐	No. of visits ☐	No. of visits ☐
_____	_____	_____
.....1 2	.....1 2	.....1 2
.....1 .....2 onto Q24	.....1 .....2 onto Q24	.....1 .....2 onto Q24
.....1 onto Q22 2	.....1 onto Q22 2	.....1 onto Q22 2

21. So when was the first time you went to ... hosp. ... as an
    outpatient about your .....?

22. How long did you have to wait for that first appointment
    at ... hosp. ...?

                            1 week or less (7 days or less) ....
        Over 1 week up to 2 weeks (8 - 14 days) ....
        Over 2 weeks up to 3 weeks (15 - 21 days) ....
        Over 3 weeks up to 4 weeks (21 - 28 days) ....
        Over 4 weeks up to 5 weeks ....
        Over 5 weeks up to 6 weeks ....
        Over 6 weeks (specify no. of weeks) ....

23. Did you mind waiting that long for the appointment or didn't
    it really matter that much?

                                    Minded waiting ....
                                    Didn't really matter ....

IF MINDED WAITING (1)

(a) Why did you mind having to wait for an appointment?

        0

CONDITION A	CONDITION B	CONDITION C
No. of visits ▢	No. of visits ▢	No. of visits ▢
before 1975 .....1 onto Q24	before 1975 .....1 onto Q24	before 1975 .....1 onto Q24
1975 2	1975 2	1975 2
1976 3	1976 3	1976 3
................1 onto Q24	................1 onto Q24	................1 onto Q24
................2	2	2
................3	3	................3.
................4	4	4
................5	5	5
................6	6	6
specify_____7	specify _____7	specify _____7
................1 ask (a)	................1 ask (a)	................1 ask (a)
................2	2	2

TO ALL WITH MORE THAN ONE VISIT IN REF. PERIOD

24. Who first referred you to ... hosp. ... about your .....?

GP, family doctor ....

Private consultant or specialist ....

O/P dept at another hospital ....

Referred after spell as in-patient ......

Casualty, accident, emergency ....

Other (specify) ....

25. Apart from the ..... visit(s) you made in ... ref months ... 197 ,
    have you had to go to ... hosp. ... since then about your ...?

Yes, had to go again ....

No that was last/only visit ....

IF YES, HAD TO GO AGAIN (1)

(a) Are you still going to ... hosp. ... about your
    ....., or have you finished going now?

Still going ....

Finished going ....

(b) So when was your last appointment at ... hosp. ...
    for your .....?

specify: Month

                Year

CONDITION A	CONDITION B	CONDITION C
No. of visits [ ]	No. of visits [ ]	No. of visits [ ]
.....1	1	1
.....2	2	2
.....3	3	3
.....4	4	4
.....5	5	5
.....6	6	6
.....1 ask (a) AND (b) .....2 go back to Q17 for details of condition B. If no cond. B go onto Q26	.....1 ask (a) AND (b) .....2 go back to Q17 for details of condition C. If no cond. C go onto Q26	.....1 ask (a) AND (b) .....2 go onto Q26
.....1 ⎱ .....2 ⎰ ask (b)	.....1 ⎱ .....2 ⎰ ask (b)	.....1 ⎱ .....2 ⎰ ask (b)
mnth [ ][ ] go back to Q17 for details of condition B. yr [7][ ] If no cond. B go onto Q26.	mnth [ ][ ] go back to Q17 for details of condition C. yr [7][ ] If no cond. C go onto Q26.	mnth [ ][ ] go onto Q26 yr [7][ ]

151

REST OF SCHEDULE REFERS ONLY TO VISITS TO
HOSPITAL FOR CONDITION A.

INTRODUCE AND EXPLAIN THAT ALL Q's NOW REFER
TO VISIT(S) FOR CONDITION A.

Interviewer to code:

Total number of visits for condition A:

only one 1

more than one 2

TRANSPORT TO THE HOSPITAL

26. How did you get to the hospital, did the
hospital send an ambulance or hospital car
for you, or did you make your own way there?

PROMPT AS NECESSARY	Always went by hospital transport	1
	Sometimes went by hospital transport ...	2
	Always made own way there	3

27. Can I check was there ever any occasion
when hospital transport was arranged for
you, but it completely failed to pick you
up?

Yes, specify no. of times⟶ [ ] ⟵ ask Q28

No, never happened 0

if coded 1 at Q26 onto Q34
if coded 2 or 3 at Q26 onto Q31

152

28. Did they let you know beforehand that you
would have to make your own way to the
hospital, or not?

PROMPT AS NECESSARY	Yes, always	1
	Yes, sometimes	2
	No	3

29. And did anyone explain to you at anytime what
had happened to the transport that should have
taken you to the hospital?

PROMPT AS NECESSARY	Yes, always explained	1
	Yes, sometimes explained .	2
	No, not explained	3

CHECK: IF INFORMANT ALWAYS WENT TO HOSPITAL
BY HOSPITAL TRANSPORT (Q26 coded 1) GO ONTO
GREEN SECTION (Q34)
OTHERS ASK Q30

30. Did you manage to make other arrangements to get
to the hospital or did it mean that you had to
miss your appointment completely for that
day?

Always made other arrangements	1	
(sometimes) Missed appointment completely	2	ask (a)

IF (SOMETIMES) MISSED APPOINTMENT COMPLETELY (2)

(a) Can I just check, how many
appointments did you miss completely
because the hospital transport failed
to pick you up?

specify number ———————▶ ☐

153

31. (On the occasions when you made your own way there)
    How did you (usually) get to the hospital; did you
    walk there, go by bus, or what?

	SINGLE CODE ONLY: Walked all the way	1
	Private car	2
CODE ALL	Hired car/taxi	3
THAT APPLY	Bus, train, tube	4
	Other (specify)	5

32. And about how long did it (usually) take you to
    get there?

About 15 (1 - 22) mins ..	1
About 30 (23 - 37) mins .	2
About 45 (38 - 50) mins .	3
About 1 hour or longer (51 mins or more) ...... Specify _____	4

33. Would you have preferred the hospital to have
    (always) laid on transport to get you there, or wasn't
    it (always) necessary?

Would have preferred hospital transport	1	ask (a)
Not necessary	2	see instruction below

IF WOULD HAVE PREFERRED HOSPITAL TRANSPORT (1)

(a) Why would you have preferred the hospital to
    have (always) laid on transport to get you
    there?

0

CHECK BACK TO Q26:

   IF ALWAYS MADE OWN WAY TO HOSPITAL (coded 3)
   SKIP GREEN SECTION AND GO ONTO Q51

   OTHERS WHO (SOMETIMES) WENT BY HOSPITAL TRANSPORT
   (coded 1 or 2) ONTO GREEN SECTION Q34

154

GREEN SECTION APPLIES ONLY TO THOSE GOING BY
HOSPITAL TRANSPORT (Q26 code 1 or 2)

34. Can I check, you said that the hospital sent an ambulance
    for you, was the hospital transport laid on by prior
    arrangement, or did you only ever go by ambulance
    when you were an emergency or accident case?

    Always OR sometimes laid on by prior arrangement   1

    Only ever went by ambulance when accident/emergency ...   2   onto Q48

35. (On the occasions when they laid on transport
    for you)

    What sort of transport did the hospital (usually)
    send for you?

    | | Ambulance - lying down or stretcher | 1 |
    | PROMPT AS NECESSARY | Ambulance - sitting or wheelchair.. | 2 |
    | | A hospital car .... | 3 |

36. Who first arranged for hospital transport to be
    laid on for you; was it ...

    | | the hospital .... | 1 |
    | RUNNING PROMPT | your own family doctor ..... | 2 |
    | | or someone else (specify)? .... | 3 |

37. Were you (usually) given a specific time when the
    ambulance/car would pick you up?

    Yes ...   1

    No ....   A   ask (a)

    IF NO (A)

    (a) Did you find this inconvenient, or
        didn't it really matter that much?

    Yes, it was inconvenient .   2

    No, didn't really matter .   3   onto Q41

38. Did the ambulance/car (usually) come at about the
    time it was supposed to?

    Yes ...   1   onto Q41

    No   2

39. Was it (usually) early or was it (usually) late?

Early ...	1	ask (a)
Late	2	ask (b)
spontaneous: sometimes early, sometimes late ..	3	

IF EARLY (1)

(a) About how early did it (usually) come?

specify no. of minutes ⟶ ☐☐☐

IF LATE (2)

(b) About how late did it (usually) come?

specify no. of minutes ⟶ ☐☐☐

40. Did it matter to you that it (usually) failed
to come at about the right time, or didn't
it really matter that much?

Yes, it mattered	1
No, didn't really matter	2

41. Did the ambulance/car (usually) have to pick
up other patients after you on the way to the
hospital or not?

Yes, picked up other patients	1	onto Q43
No	2	

42. Can I just check, when you got to the hospital,
were you (usually) the only patient in the
ambulance/car, or were there (usually) other patients
as well?

Only informant	1	onto Q45
Other patients as well .	2	

43. Did the ambulance/car (usually) have to go out
of its way to pick up any of these other patients,
or did they all live more or less on the way to
the hospital?

Had to go out of its way	A	ask (a)
Lived on way to hospital	1	

IF HAD TO GO OUT OF ITS WAY (A)

(a) On the whole did you quite enjoy the
trip around or would you have preferred
to have gone straight to the hospital?

Quite enjoyed the trip around	2
Preferred to have gone straight to hospital	3

156

44. Before you were picked up, did you (usually)
know there were other patients to be collected
after you, or not?

Yes, knew there were other patients to be collected ..	1	
No, didn't know	2	

45. How long did it (usually) take you to get
to the hospital by ambulance/hospital car?

About 15 (1-22) mins	1
About 30 (23-37) mins	2
About 45 (38-50) mins	3
About 1 hour or longer (51 mins or more) specify ———	4

46. Did the journey (ever), take very much longer than
you thought it would?

Yes, took longer than thought	A	ask (a)
No	1	

IF TOOK LONGER THAN THOUGHT (A)

(a) Did you find this inconvenient or
distressing or didn't it really matter?

Yes inconvenient/distressing .	2
No, didn't really matter	3

47. Bearing in mind your condition/ailment, was your
journey to hospital (usually) reasonably comfortable?

Yes	1	onto Q51
No	2	ask (a)

IF NO (2)

(a) What could have been done to have
made it more comfortable?

0

Nothing	1	
Don't know	2	onto Q51
Other (specify)	3	

onto Q51

48. What sort of ambulance did the hospital send for
you, was it a stretcher ambulance, or one you
could sit up in?

Ambulance - lying down or stretcher	1
Ambulance - sitting or wheelchair	2
SPONTANEOUS: Hospital car	3

49. How long did it take for the ambulance/car to
come?

Don't know - was unconscious, had no awareness of time	1
Can't remember	2
Less than 15 minutes	3
Other: specify no. of minutes ———	
	ask (a)

IF WAITED 15 MINS OR MORE

(a) Do you think the ambulance/car took an
unreasonable length of time to come or
not?

Yes	1
No	2

50. Bearing in mind your condition/ailment, was your
journey to hospital reasonably comfortable?

Don't know - unconscious	1	
Yes	2	
No	3	ask (a)

IF NO (3)

(a) What could have been done to make your
journey to hospital in the ambulance/car
more comfortable?

Nothing	1
Don't know	2
Other (specify) ...	3

51. How did you get back from the hospital afterwards?
    Did you go back by ambulance, or by hospital car,
    or did you make your own way back?

PROMPT AS	Always went back by hospital transport	1	onto Q55
NECESSARY	Sometimes went back by hospital transport	2	
	Always made own way back	3	

52. (On the occasions) When you made your own way
    back from hospital, did you (usually) walk back,
    get a bus, or what?

SINGLE CODE ONLY	Walked all the way ...	1
CODE ALL THAT APPLY	Private car	2
	Hired car/taxi	3
	Bus, train, tube	4
	Other (specify)	5

53. And about how long did it (usually) take
    you to get back from the hospital?

About 15 (1-22) mins	1
About 30 (23-37) mins	2
About 45 (38-50) mins	3
About 1 hour or longer (51 mins or more) specify	4

159

54. Would you have preferred the hospital to have
    (always) laid on transport back or wasn't it
    (always) necessary?

Would have preferred hospital transport	1	ask (a)
Not necessary	2	see instruction below

IF WOULD HAVE PREFERRED HOSPITAL TRANSPORT (1)

(a) Why would you have preferred the hospital
    to have (always) laid on transport back
    for you?

    0

CHECK BACK TO Q51:

IF ALWAYS MADE OWN WAY BACK FROM HOSPITAL
(coded 3) SKIP GREEN SECTION GO ONTO Q65
OTHERS WHO (SOMETIMES) WENT BACK BY
HOSPITAL TRANSPORT (coded 1 or 2) ONTO
GREEN SECTION Q55

55. (On the occasions when they laid on transport)
What sort of transport did the hospital (usually)
provide to take you back?

PROMPT AS NECESSARY	ambulance - lying down or stretcher ...	1
	ambulance - sitting or wheelchair	2
	hospital car	3

56. When you arrived at the hospital did you know that
you would be given hospital transport to take you
back, or did special arrangements (usually) have
to be made?

Knew would be given transport	1
Special arrangements..........	2

57. Were you (usually) told how long you would have
to wait after you had finished being seen before
the ambulance/car would take you back?

Yes told ...	1
No, not told	2

161

58. After you had finished being seen at the hospital
    how long did you (usually) have to wait before
    the ambulance/car left to take you back?

                          About 15 mins or less (1-22 mins)   1
                          About 30 (23-37) mins   2
                          About 45 (38-50) mins   3   ask (a)
                          About 1 hour or longer (51 mins
                            or more) specify:_____   4

    IF CODED (2)(3) or (4)

    (a) Was having to wait around for the
        ambulance/car inconvenient or
        distressing or (on the whole) didn't
        you really mind that much?

                          Yes, inconvenient/distressing ...   1
                          No, didn't really mind   2

59. Did the ambulance/car (usually) take other patients
    home, or were you (usually) the only patient in
    the ambulance/car?

                          Took other patients home   1
                          Informant was only patient   2   onto Q62

60. Were you (usually) dropped off first, or did
    some of the other patients get dropped off before
    you?

                          Informant was first   1   onto Q62
                          Other patients dropped off first .   2

61. Did the ambulance/car (usually) drop these other
    patients off more or less on your way home, or did
    it (usually) take you out of your way?

                          On the way home ..... | 1 |
                          Taken out of the way | A | ask (a)

    IF TAKEN OUT OF WAY (A)

    (a) On the whole did you quite enjoy the trip
        around, or would you have preferred to have
        gone straight back?

                          Quite enjoyed trip around .. | 2 |
                          Preferred to have gone
                            straight back .... | 3 |

62. How long did it (usually) take you to get back
    home in the ambulance/car?

                          About 15 (1-22) mins .... | 1 |
                          About 30 (23-37) mins ...... | 2 |
                          About 45 (38-50) mins ...... | 3 |
                          About 1 hour or longer (51
                            mins or more) specify: | 4 |
                          _____

63. Did the journey back (ever) take very much longer than
    you thought it would?
                          Yes, took longer than thought .... | A | ask (a)
                          No .... | 1 |

    IF YES TOOK LONGER THAN THOUGHT (A)

    (a) Did you find this inconvenient or
        distressing or didn't it really matter?

                          Yes, inconvenient or distressing .. | 1 |
                          No, didn't really matter .... | 2 |

64. Bearing in mind your condition was the journey back
from hospital (usually) reasonably comfortable?

Yes   1

No   2   ask (a)

IF NO (2)

(a) What could have been done to make the
journey back from hospital in the ambulance/
car more comfortable?

0   Nothing   1

Don't know   2

Other (specify) ..   3

164

TO ALL : FACILITIES

Introduce:

Before I go on to ask you about the facilities at the
hospital, can I check ...

65. (On your last visit to ..... about your .....)
When you arrived at the hospital which department
or clinic did you go to first?

Outpatients	1
Casualty, accident, emergency	2
X ray	3
Other (specify dept. or treatment if dept. not known)	4

[Q66 - 86 refer to facilities in this department]

66. The first time you went to the ..... dept. about
your ....., were you able to find it all right or
did you have any difficulty?

Found dept. all right	1
Had difficulty	2

67. Is the ..... department at the hospital on the
ground floor, or do you have to go up or down
to another floor to get to it?

On ground floor	1	onto Q69
On upper or lower floor ..	2	

165

68. Was there a lift that patients could use or not?

Yes	1	
No	2	ask (a)
DK	3	

IF NO (2) or DK (3)

(a) Could you manage the stairs all right
    or did you have any difficulty?

Could manage all right .	1
Had difficulty	2

69. I'd like to ask you now about the facilities provided
    for patients in the ..... department while they are
    waiting to be seen ...

    When you were there were there (usually) enough seats
    for everyone who was waiting to be seen?

Yes	1
No	2

70. And were the seats ...

	comfortable	1
RUNNING PROMPT	were they all right	2
	or, bearing in mind your condition, did you find them uncomfortable?	3	ask (a)
	SPONTANEOUS: Don't know, not used	4

IF UNCOMFORTABLE (3)

(a) Why did you find them rather
    uncomfortable?

    0

71. <u>When you were there</u>, was there (usually) enough
    room in the waiting area for everyone who had to
    be seen, or did it (often) get overcrowded?

(usually) enough room	1
(often) got overcrowded	2

72. Was the waiting area in the ..... department
    (usually) reasonably clean and tidy or not?

Yes, clean and tidy	1
No	2

73. And thinking generally about the appearance of
    the waiting area in the ..... department, would
    you say that it was ...

a bright and cheerful place to wait in ..	1
that it was all right	2
RUNNING PROMPT that it was a bit drab and depressing ...	3
or didn't you take that much notice of its appearance?	4

74. Were there (usually) magazines or newspapers for you
    to look at while you were waiting to be seen?

Yes ...	1	
No	A	ask (a)
SPONTANEOUS: Can't remember	2	

IF NO (A)

(a) Would you have liked something to read or
    look at while you were waiting or weren't
    you really bothered?

Yes, would have liked something to read	3
No, not really bothered	4

167

TO ALL PROXIES FOR CHILD PATIENTS

(Others go onto Q76)

75. Was there anything to keep children
    occupied while they were waiting to
    be seen?

                     SINGLE CODE ONLY: No, nothing   1   ask (a)

         PROMPT AS   Yes, books/comics ...   2
         NECESSARY AND   Yes, toys, games   3
         CODE ALL THAT
         APPLY   Yes, other (specify)   4

IF NO, NOTHING PROVIDED (1)

(a) Would it have helped if there
    had been some comics or toys or
    wasn't ... child ... really bothered?

                         Yes, would have helped   1
                         No, not really bothered   2

TO ALL

76. Was there anywhere either in the ..... department, or
    nearby to get a cup of tea or something to eat while
    waiting to be seen?

                     Yes, somewhere to get tea and/
                         or food   1
                     No   2   onto Q79
                     Don't know   3

168

77. Where could you get tea or coffee from ... was there
a refreshment bar, a machine, a trolley or what?

Refreshment bar	A	ask (a)
Machine	1	
Trolley	2	onto Q78
Other (specify)	3	

IF REFRESHMENT BAR (A)

(a) Was the refreshment bar (usually) open
while you were there?

Yes (incl. for only some of the time)	4
No, not at all	5

78. Would people have any difficulty finding where to go
for a cup of tea, or is it quite easy to find?

People would have difficulty	1	onto Q80
Quite easy to find	2	

79. (Generally) would you have liked to have been able to
get something to eat or drink while waiting,
or weren't you really bothered?

Would have liked refreshment	1
Not really bothered	2
SPONTANEOUS: Couldn't eat/drink because of condition .	3

80. Was there a public telephone either in the .....
department or nearby that patients could use if they
wanted to do so?

Yes	A	ask (a)
No	1	
Don't know ...	2	

IF YES (A)
(a) Would people have any difficulty finding where the
telephone was, or is it quite easy to find?

Would have difficulty .	3	ontoQ81
Quite easy to find	4	

169

81. Would it have put your mind at rest if there had
    been a public telephone, or weren't you really
    bothered?

                    Yes, would have set mind at rest   1

                    No, not really bothered   2

82. While you were at the ..... department, did you
    (ever) use the toilet facilities?

                            Yes used ....   A   ask (a)(b)

                            No, not used   1   onto Q83

    IF YES USED (A)

    (a) Was the toilet (usually) clean or not?

                            Yes   2
                            No   3

    (b) Was there (usually) toilet paper in the cubicle?

                            Yes   1
                            No   2
            SPONTANEOUS: Can't remember   3

83. And was there somewhere to wash and dry your
    hands?

                            Yes   1
                            No   2
            SPONTANEOUS: Can't remember   3

84. Is the toilet quite easy to find, or do you think
    people might have difficulty in finding it?

                    Quite easy to find   1
                                                          onto Q86
                    Might have difficulty   2

85. Can I check, was that because you didn't (ever)
    need to use the toilet facilities, or for some other
    reason?

	Didn't need to use toilet	1
	Thought might miss turn	2
CODE ALL	Didn't like using "public"	
THAT APPLY	toilets	3
	Couldn't find patients toilet ..	4
	Other (specify)	5

86. I shall be asking you next about how long you had
    to wait to be seen, but apart from that and
    bearing in mind your condition/ailment ...

    Did you find the waiting area in the ..... department
    ...

	very comfortable	1
RUNNING	all right	2
PROMPT	rather uncomfortable	3
	or very uncomfortable?	4

171

WAITING TO SEE THE DOCTOR

[If only ever made one visit for condition A and
that was without an appointment (ie casualty
etc) go onto Q94.]

Others - introduce

87. I'd now like to ask you about your appointment(s)
at the hospital ...

When appointments were made for you to attend
the ..... department did you usually have a say
in fixing the most convenient time or not?

Yes, had a say .	1	
No	A	ask (a)

IF NO (A)

(a) Would you have preferred your appointments
to be fixed for a different time, or were
they usually all right for you?

Preferred a different time	2	ask (i)
Usually all right	3	

IF PREFERRED A DIFFERENT TIME (2)

(i) Why is that?

0

88. Were your appointments (usually) fixed for a specific
time or were you (usually) asked to go along between
certain times?

Fixed for a specific time	1	
Between certain times	2	onto Q94

89. Did you think that you were the only patient being
given that appointment time, or did you think that
(sometimes) other patients were also being told to
come along at that time?

Individual appointment time	1
Others being told same time	2
SPONTANEOUS:Don't know, never thought about it	3

172

90. Did you (usually) arrive within 5 or 10 minutes either way of your appointment time, or were you (usually) earlier than that?

Arrived within 5 or 10 minutes ...	1	
Earlier than that	2	ask (a)
SPONTANEOUS: (Usually) Late	3	

IF EARLIER THAN THAT (2)

(a) Why did you usually get there early?

Thought might be seen <u>before appt. time</u>	1	onto Q93
Thought would be "first in the queue"..	2	
CODE ALL THAT APPLY Transport gets there early – no option	3	
Like to leave plenty of time	4	
Other (specify)	5	

0

Interviewer: Don't forget to delete the verbatim you put in the precodes

91. Did you (usually) expect to be seen within 5 or 10 minutes of your appointment time, or did you (usually) expect to have to wait longer than that?

Expected to be seen within 5 or 10 minutes	1	onto Q93
Expected to have to wait longer	2	

173

92 How long after your appointment time
    did you (usually) expect to have to wait?

                    SPONTANEOUS: No idea   0   onto Q93

                    About 15 (13-22) minutes.............   1   ⌉
                    About 30 (23-37) minutes.............   2
                                                                      ask (a)
                    About 45 (38-50) minutes.............   3 .
                    About 1 hour or longer (51 minutes or
                             more) specify: 4   ⌋

    IF 15 MINUTES OR LONGER (CODES 1-4)
    (a) What made you think you would have
    to wait that long?

        0

93 (Thinking specifically about the last time
    you went to.......hosp..... about your....)
    Were you actually seen within 5 or 10
    minutes of your appointment time or did you
    have to wait longer than that?

                    Seen within 5 or 10 minutes (incl.
                             seen early)   1   onto Q100
                    Waited longer than that..............   2   ask (a)

    IF WAITED LONGER THAN THAT(2)
    (a) So how long after your appointment
    time was it before you were seen?

                    About 15 (13-22) minutes.............   1   ⌉
                    About 30 (23-37) minutes.............   2   onto Q96
                    About 45 (38-50) minutes.............   3
                    About 1 hour or longer (51 minutes
                             or more) specify: 4   ⌋

174

94 When you got to the hospital how long
    did you (usually) think you would have
    to wait before you would be seen (by
    a doctor)?

                    Unconscious, dazed - no idea........   0
                                                                    onto Q95
                    Conscious but no idea................   9

                    About 5 or 10 (1-12) minutes........   1

                    About 15 (13-22) minutes............   2

                    About 30 (23-37) minutes............   3

                    About 45 (38-50) minutes............   4   ask (a)

                    About 1 hour or longer (51 minutes
                        or more) specify:..............   5

IF 15 MINUTES OR LONGER (CODES 2-5)
(a) What made you think you would have
to wait that long?

     0

95 (Thinking specifically about the last
    time you went to...hosp... about your......)

    How long was it before you were actually
    seen by a doctor?

                    Unconscious, dazed - don't know......   0
                                                                    onto Q100
                    About 5 or 10 (1-12) minutes (incl.
                                    immediately)........   1

                    About 15 (13-22) minutes............   2

                    About 30 (23-37) minutes............   3
                                                                    ask Q96
                    About 45 (38-50) minutes............   4

                    About 1 hour or longer (51 minutes or
                                    more) specify: 5

175

TO ALL WHO WAITED 'ABOUT 15 MINUTES' OR LONGER
TO BE SEEN

96 Were you told why it was that you
    had to wait to be seen?

                        Yes, told.............   1
                        No, not told..........   2

97 Do you personally think that this was an unreasonable time
    to wait or not?

                        Yes, unreasonable...........   1   ask (a)
                        No, not unreasonable........   2

    IF YES UNREASONABLE (1)
    (a) Why was that?

        ()

98 Were you told how long you might
    have to wait to be seen when you got to the hospital?

                        Yes, told.............   1   onto Q100
                        No, not told..........   2

176

99. Would it have helped if, when you arrived
    at the hospital, you had been told how
    long you might have to wait, or not?

                              Yes, would have helped ....   A   ask (a)

                              No   1   onto Q100

    IF YES WOULD HAVE HELPED (A)
    (a) Did you ask how long you might have
    to wait to be seen?

                              Yes, asked   2
                              No did not ask ,..........   3   ask (i)

          IF NO, DID NOT ASK (3)
          (i) Why didn't you ask?

    TO ALL
100. (Thinking about your last visit to hospital)....
     After you had been seen in the ... dept., did you
     get sent on to any other department or clinic in
     the hospital?

                              Yes .. ..,   A

                              No ....,   1   onto Q102

     If YES (A)
     (a) Did you feel you had to wait an unreasonable
     length of time before being seen in any of these
     other departments or not?

                              Yes waited unreasonable time   2   ask (i)and(ii)
                              No   3

          If YES WAITED UNREASONABLE TIME (2)
          (i) In which department was that?

     ⌈ Specify treatment   ⌉
     ⌊ if dept not known   ⌋

          (ii) How long did you have to wait there before
          you were seen?
                              About 1 hr or longer (51 mins
                                       or more)...............   1
                              About 45 (38 - 50) mins.......   2
                              About 30 (23 - 37) mins   3
                              About 15 (13 - 22) mins.......   4
                              Less than that...............   5

101. And still thinking about that (last) visit, were
     you sent on to any other department or clinic
     where the conditions in the waiting room were
     really inadequate?

                                          Yes   1   ask (a)(b)

                                          No   2

        If YES (1)
        (a) Which department was that?

        ⎡ Specify treatment ⎤
        ⎣ if dept. not known ⎦

        (b) What in particular was inadequate?

            ()

102. Just thinking very generally now,.....
     if you have to go to hospital as an
     outpatient would you prefer to be given
     a specific appointment time, or would
     you prefer to be told to go along at
     any time between certain hours?

                     Prefer specific appointment time ..   1

                     Prefer to go between certain times   2   onto Q104

         SPONTANEOUS·   No preference   3   onto Q105

103. Why do you prefer to be given a specific
     appointment time, rather than being told
     to go along at any time between certain
     hours?

     0

                         onto Q105

_____

104. Why do you prefer _not_ to have
     a specific appointment time?

     ∩

_____

105. And still thinking very generally, do you
     personally think that on the whole the hospital
     appointment system is.........................

            RUNNING   mainly for the benefit of
            PROMPT   the doctors...................   1

                             or mainly for the benefit of
                             the patients?   2

       SPONTANEOUS ONLY   "50/50"   3

106. Thinking back to when you were waiting to be dealt
    with in the ..... dept, how did you know when it
    was your turn to go in?

Informant was (always) only
    patient there 0   onto Q110

Other answers (specify) ... 1

107. Was this a satisfactory way of letting you know
    or could it have been improved in some way?

Satisfactory 1

Could be improved 2   ask (a)

IF COULD BE IMPROVED (2)

(a) How could it have been improved?

Don't know, no idea 1

Other (specify) 2

108. When you went in to be seen could other patients (usually)
    overhear what was being said to you, or not?

Yes, other patients could hear 1   ask (a)(b)

No, other patients could not hear . 2

Don't know 3

IF YES (1)

(a) Did this bother you ...

quite a lot 1

only a little 2

RUNNING
PROMPT   or didn't it really bother you
            at all? 3

(b) Did it (ever) bother you overhearing
    what was being said to other patients?

Yes 1

No 2

Couldn't hear/no other patients 3

109. And when you were being treated could you (usually) be seen by other patients or not?

Yes could be seen	1	ask (a)(b)
No, could not be seen	2	
Don't know	3	

IF YES (1)

(a) Did this bother you ...

	quite a lot	1
RUNNING	only a little	2
PROMPT	or didn't it really bother you at all?	3

(b) Did seeing other patients being treated (ever) bother you or not?

Yes	1
No	2
Couldn't see/no other patients	3

110. On (any of) your visits to ... hosp. ... about your ... cond. ... were there (ever) any medical students present while you were being treated or examined?

Yes	1	
No	2	onto Q112

111. Were you asked if you agreed to their being present or not?

Yes (incl. sometimes) ...	1	
No, never	A	ask (a)(b)
Can't remember	2	

IF NO, NEVER (A)

(a) Did you mind not being asked, or weren't you really bothered?

Yes, minded	3
Not really bothered	4

(b) And did you mind the medical students being there, or didn't it really worry you?

Yes, minded	1
No, not worried	2

112. Did you (ever) have to undress to be treated
or examined?

Yes	A	ask (a)
No	1	

IF YES (A)

(a) Were the arrangements for undressing
and getting dressed again (usually)
satisfactory?

Yes, satisfactory ...	2	
No, unsatisfactory ..	3	ask (i)

IF NO (3)

(i) Why were they unsatisfactory?

0

113. Did the doctors at the hospital (always) tell you
enough about how you were getting on, or what you
had to have done, or did you (ever) want to know
more?

(Always) Told enough	1	onto Q116
Wanted to know more	2	

114 Did you feel that you could ask the doctors to tell
you what you wanted to know, or not?

	Yes, could ask all doctors	1	
PROMPT AS NECESSARY	Yes, could ask only some doctors, not others	2	ask (a)
	No, could not ask any doctors ..	3	

IF YES COULD ASK ALL OR SOME DOCTORS (1) OR (2)

(a) When you asked the doctors what you
wanted to know, did you generally get
a satisfactory answer?

Yes	1	
No	2	onto Q116
Never asked any questions	3	

182

115. Why did you feel that you couldn't ask the doctors what you wanted to know?

    0

Don't know/just didn't ask	1
Other (specify)	2

116. Did you always understand what the doctors told you about your condition and treatment, or would you sometimes have liked it explained in everyday language?

Understood	1	
Would have liked it explained .	A	ask (a)

IF WOULD LIKE IT EXPLAINED (A)

(a) Did you (ever) ask any other doctor or nurse at the hospital to explain what had been said to you?

Yes	2
No	3

117. <u>Apart from using medical terms</u>, did you ever have any difficulty in simply understanding what any of the doctors were saying?

Yes, had difficulty .	1	ask (a)
No, no difficulty ...	2	

IF YES HAD DIFFICULTY (1)

(a) What was the difficulty?

    0

CHECK: if informant didn't understand what doctor said <u>either</u> at Q116 (coded A) <u>or</u> at Q117 (coded 1) ask Q118 (Others go onto Q119)

118. How did you personally feel about not always understanding what the doctors were saying? Were you ...

	Not really bothered ...	1
RUNNING PROMPT	Worried or upset by it	2
	or were you embarrassed? .	3

⌈ Qs 119 - 121 refer to items of treatment A-H as
specified in grid below, and answers to these
questions are coded in the grid. ⌋

Introduce: Can we talk now about the treatment you had as an
outpatient while you were at hospital.

119. (On any of the visits you made to ... hosp. ... about
your ... cond. A ...).

Did you (ever) have ..... INDIVIDUALLY PROMPT ITEMS A-H
AND CODE BELOW Yes = 1
No = 2

		Q119	
		YES	NO
A	a blood sample taken or a blood test?	.. 1	2...
B	any injections?	.. 1	2...
C	X-rays?	.. 1	2...
D	physiotherapy?	.. 1	2...
E	give a water or urine specimen while you were at the hospital?...	.. 1	2...
F	a general anaesthetic - (being put to sleep for a short while)?...	.. 1	2...
G	stitches or clips or have them removed?	.. 1.............	2...
H	dressings done, changed or removed?	.. 1.............	2...

⌈ Ask Q120 for each item coded Yes (1) except G & H
if Q120 DNA see instruction above Q121 ⌋

120. Thinking about when you had (... the blood sample taken ...)
were you told enough about why it was necessary?

RING CODES IN GRID   Yes, told enough   = 3
No, not told enough = 4

For each item coded (4) - NO, NOT TOLD ENOUGH ask (a)

(a) Were you bothered by this or not?

RING CODES IN GRID   Yes, bothered   = 5
No, not bothered = 6

184

If <u>any</u> item coded Yes (1) at Q119 ask Q121
if <u>no</u> item coded Yes (1) go to Q123

121. You said you had ..... [read out items of treatment received] were any of these things particularly unpleasant or not?

<u>EITHER</u> CODE HERE: none of the treatment was unpleasant ...   0

<u>OR</u> RING CODE 7 BELOW for each item of treatment that was unpleasant

For each item coded (7) - UNPLEASANT ask (a)

(a) Could anything have been done to make it less unpleasant?

RING CODES BELOW: Yes, something could be done = 8

No, nothing could be done   = 9

Q120		Q120(a)		Q121	Q121(a)	
YES - told enough	N O - not told enough	YES bothered	NO - not bothered	UN- PLEASANT	YES	NO
3	4	..... 5	6	..... 7	.... 8	9
3 ...,...............	4	..... 5	6	..... 7	.... 8	9
3	4	..... 5	6	..... 7	.... 8	9
3	4	..... 5	6	..... 7	.... 8	9
3	4	..... 5	6	..... 7	.... 8	9
3	4	..... 5 ,.......	6 ,....	..... 7	.... 8	9
				..... 7	..... 8	9
				..... 7	..... 8	9

REMEMBER Q121 IS ABOVE GRID

185

Q122 applies only to WOMEN WHO GAVE A URINE SPECIMEN AT
THE HOSPITAL - Q119 item E coded 1 (others see Q123)

122. You said that you had to give a specimen of your
water while you were at the hospital ...
Could you manage this all right, or were there (ever)
any problems or difficulties in providing a specimen?

Managed all right 1

Had problems/difficulties 2   ask (a)

IF HAD PROBLEMS/DIFFICULTY (2)

(a) What was the trouble?

    0

TO ALL WHO MADE ONLY ONE VISIT FOR CONDITION A
(Others go onto Q125)

123. On that particular visit to ..... how long were
you at the hospital in all?

Less than 30 mins 1

30 mins less than 1 hour 2

1 hr less than 1½ hours 3

1½ hours less than 2 hours 4

2 hours less than 2½ hours 5

2½ hours less than 3 hours 6

3 hours and over (specify) 7

_____

124. Before you went, did you expect to be there ...

much longer than you were 1

about that long 2

RUNNING
PROMPT   or did you expect to be dealt with
more quickly? 3   onto Q127

SPONTANEOUS: No idea of what to expect 4

125. On your last visit to ..... about your ..... how long
     were you at the hospital in all?

Less than 30 mins	1	
30 mins less than 1 hour	2	
1 hour less than 1½ hours ...	3	
1½ hours less than 2 hours ..	4	
2 hours less than 2½ hours ..	5	
2½ hours less than 3 hours ..	6	
3 hours and over (specify) _____	7	

126. Were you usually there ...

much longer than that	1	ask (a)
about that long	2	
RUNNING PROMPT or were you usually dealt with more quickly than on your last visit	3	ask (a)
SPONTANEOUS: Can't say - each visit very different	4	

IF CODED (1) OR (3)

(a) How long were you usually at the
    hospital?

Less than 30 mins	1
30 mins less than 1 hour	2
1 hour less than 1½ hours ...	3
1½ hours less than 2 hours ..	4
2 hours less than 2½ hours ..	5
2½ hours less than 3 hours ..	6
3 hours and over (specify) _____	7

TO ALL

127. Bearing in mind what was done while you were at
hospital, do you think that overall you (usually) spent
a reasonable amount of time at the hospital, do
you think you were (usually) dealt with too quickly,
or do you think you were (usually) there too long?

Spent a reasonable amount of time there 1

Dealt with too quickly 2   onto Q129

There too long 3

SPONTANEOUS: Sometimes too quick/sometimes too long 4

128. Was there any stage in your treatment when you felt
that more time should have been spent on you, or were
you satisfied that enough time had been taken over
your case?

More time should have been spent ... 1

Satisfied with time taken 2   onto Q130

129. Which stage in your case or treatment do you
think they should have taken more time over?

All stages 1

Other (specify) 2

188

130. I'd now like to ask you briefly about how you felt
     about the staff you met while you were an out-patient
     at ..... Thinking about the nurses you met while you
     were there, did you find that ...

RUNNING PROMPT	all of them were considerate	1
	that most of them were considerate	2
	or that only a few of them were considerate?	3
SPONTANEOUS:	not met enough/any - can't say	4

131. And how about medical staff, people like
     physiotherapists, radiographers and dieticians,
     did you find that ...

RUNNING PROMPT	all of them were nice to you	1
	that most of them were nice to you	2
	or that only a few of them were nice to you?	3
SPONTANEOUS:	not met enough/any - can't say	4

132. And how about the non-medical staff at the
     hospital - the porters, receptionists and
     orderlies; were ...

RUNNING PROMPT	all of them helpful	1
	most of them helpful	2
	or only a few of them helpful?	3
SPONTANEOUS:	not met enough/any - can't say	4

133. We've talked now about many aspects of your
     visit(s) to hospital, so thinking of your own
     experience, would you personally say that on
     the whole the hospital service for outpatients
     is ...

	very good	1
RUNNING PROMPT	good	2
	has its faults	3
	or is poor?	4

189

134. Apart from your visit(s) to ... hosp. ... as an outpatient,
     have you ever been in ... hosp. ... as an inpatient
     overnight or longer in connection with ... cond. A ...?

Yes	1	
No	2	onto Q141

135. How many times have you been into hospital
     as an inpatient in connection with your
     ... cond. A ... <u>since January 1975?</u>

None	0	onto Q141
Specify number ————		

136. And how many nights were you in hospital on
     that (the last) occasion?

overnight	1	
2 nights	2	onto Q140
3 - 5	3	
6 - 7	4	
8 - 14	5	
15 - 21	6	
over 3 weeks (specify to nearest week) _____	7	

137. (Thinking about your last spell in hospital ...)
On that occasion what did you think about the
arrangements for your admission, were you ...

	very satisfied	1	
RUNNING PROMPT	satisfied	2	
	or could they have been improved?	3	ask (a)

IF COULD HAVE BEEN IMPROVED (3)

(a) How could they have been improved?

0

138. And how about the arrangements made for discharging
you from hospital, were you ...

	very satisfied	1	
RUNNING PROMPT	satisfied	2	
	or could they have been improved?.....	3	ask (a)

IF COULD HAVE BEEN IMPROVED (3)

(a) How could they have been improved?

0

139. Are there any (other) improvements that you would
     like to suggest which could have made your stay
     in hospital on that (last) occasion more
     agreeable?

No, nothing ..	0
Yes (specify)	1

0

140. Would you personally say, from your own experience
     that overall the hospital service <u>for inpatients</u>
     is ...

	very good	1
RUNNING	good	2
PROMPT	has its faults ...	3
	or is poor?..........	4

192

CLASSIFICATION, OCCUPATION, INDUSTRY AND INCOME

(If informant is under 16 collect all information from parent)

Introduce:

141. HOUSEHOLD COMPOSITION

RELATIONSHIP TO OUTPATIENT		HOH	H' WIFE	SEX		AGE LAST BIRTH-DAY	MARITAL STATUS			WORKING STATUS			
	Office use			M	F		M	S	Wid Sep Div	FULL TIME (over 30)	PART TIME (over 10-30)	UN-EMPLOYED	NOT WORKING
PATIENT		1	2	1	2		1	2	3	1	2	3	4
		1	2	1	2		1	2	3	1	2	3	4
		1	2	1	2		1	2	3	1	2	3	4
		1	2	1	2		1	2	3	1	2	3	4
		1	2	1	2		1	2	3	1	2	3	4
		1	2	1	2		1	2	3	1	2	3	4
		1	2	1	2		1	2	3	1	2	3	4
		1	2	1	2		1	2	3	1	2	3	4
		1	2	1	2		1	2	3	1	2	3	4
		1	2	1	2		1	2	3	1	2	3	4
		1	2	1	2		1	2	3	1	2	3	4

Number of persons in household ....

IF PATIENT IS AGED 16 OR OVER AND NOT WORKING ASK Q141(a)

141. (a) Are you ...

	retired	1
PROMPT AS NECESSARY	permanently sick/disabled	2
	temp. off-sick - no job to return to	3
	housewife	4
CODE FIRST THAT APPLIES	at school	5
	in other full-time education?	6

142. PATIENT'S OCCUPATION OR IF
     RETIRED LAST MAIN OCCUPATION

     DNA Patient aged under 16
          or never worked ...... | X onto
                                  | Q144

     What is your job? What
     do you actually do?

144. HOH'S OCCUPATION OR IF
     RETIRED LAST MAIN
     OCCUPATION

     DNA Patient is HOH .... | X onto Q146

     What is your
     (..HOH's) job?
     What does he actually
     do?

143. PATIENT'S INDUSTRY

     What does the firm/
     organisation you work for
     actually make or do?

                  Are you an employee . | 1
                  or self-employed? ... | 2

     If manager,superintendent,
     self-employed:

     How many people work in the
     establishment?

                        1-24 .. | X
                        25 + .. | Y

145. HOH'S INDUSTRY

     What does the firm/
     organisation he works
     for actually make or do?

                  Is he an employee . | 1
                  or self-employed? . | 2

     If manager,
     superintendent, self-
     employed:

     How many people work in
     the establishment?

                        1-24 .. | X
                        25 + .. | Y

INCOME:

146. Please could you look at this card (HAND OVER INCOME
CARD) and tell me into which of the 8 groups your
own income falls. This includes the income from all
sources, after income tax, National Insurance and other
deductions have been taken off.

CODE BELOW AND THEN REPEAT QUESTION FOR HOH's INCOME

Per week	Annual	Patient	HOH
Nil	Nil	1	1
up to £10	up to £520	2	2
over £10 - £20	over £520 - £1040 ...	3	3
over £20 - £40	over £1040 - £2080 ..	4	4
over £40 - £60	over £2080 - £3120 ..	5	5
over £60 - £80	over £3120 - £4160 ..	6	6
over £80 - £100	over £4160 - £5200 ..	7	7
over £100	over £5200	8	8
If patient is HOH ring code		9	
Don't know			9
Refused/not asked - code and write in reason		0	0

CHECK: If patient AND/OR HOH is earning less than
£2080 (codes 1 - 4) ask Q147
(If both patient AND HOH are earning over £2080 go onto Q148)

147. Could I check, are you (is your ..HOH ..)
currently receiving supplementary benefit?

	Patient	HOH
Yes, is receiving supp. benefit....	1	1
No	2	2
Don't know		3
If patient is HOH ring code	3	

148. Finally apart from the things we've discussed already
is there anything else that you would like to say
about your visit(s) to ... hosp. ... as an
<u>outpatient</u> for your... cond. ...?

No 1

Yes (specify)   2

┌─────────────────────────────────────┐
│ THANK INFORMANT FOR CO-OPERATION   │
│ LEAVE LEAFLET   │
└─────────────────────────────────────┘

PATIENTS ATTITUDES TO THE HOSPITAL SERVICE   S1107 Mainstage
INPATIENT QUESTIONNAIRE : IN CONFIDENCE

Serial number [ ][ ][ ][ ][ ]

(i)   Interviewers name _____

(ii) Authorisation number _____

(iii) Date of interview _____/_____/197_____

(iv) Interview with: sampled person aged 14 or over......... 1

                        proxy taken for sampled person under
                        14 years 2

                        relationship of proxy (specify)
                        _____

Copy from sampling sheet before interview:

(a) Date of GHS interview   [ ][ ]   [ ][ ] /197 [ ]
                             day   month   year

(b) Inpatient details:

SEX	
M	F
1	2

AGE	

(c) Inpatient spells:

	1st SPELL	2nd SPELL	3rd SPELL	4th SPELL
(i) Month				
(ii) Year	197 [ ]	197 [ ]	197 [ ]	197 [ ]
(iii) Department:				
Medical/surgical ..	 1	 1	 1	 1
Maternity	 2	 2	 2	 2
Other	 3	 3	 3	 3

197

1. Can I start by asking you, from your own experience
   as an inpatient would you personally say that
   on the whole the hospital service for inpatients is ...

	very good	1
RUNNING	good	2
PROMPT	has its faults	3
	or is poor?..............	4

2. I believe you went into hospital in _____ 197_,
   (and again in _____ 197_)
   Have you been back into hospital as an inpatient
   at all since then?

Yes, been inpatient again .	1	
No, no further inpatient experience .	2	onto Q5

3. When was the last time you went in?

   month ....

   year 7

4. And how long were you in hospital on that last
   occasion?

   [Check for no of nights]

overnight	1
2 nights	2
3-5 nights	3
6-7 nights	4
8-14 nights	5
15-21 nights	6
over 3 weeks (specify to nearest week) _____	7

198

5. We are particularly interested in the spell you had in
   hospital in _____/197 ....

   [START WITH FIRST (EARLIEST) SPELL IN REFERENCE PERIOD]

   When you went into hospital on that occasion what
   was it for?

   ⌈ Give full details   ⌉   Maternity (normal delivery) ...   1
   | of condition, symptoms, |
   ⌊ treatment   ⌋

   Condition

   A

_____

6. What was the name of the hospital you were in?

                    specify: _____

_____

199

7. And were you in hospital as a National Health Service patient or as a private patient?

National Health Service ...	A	ask (a)
Private patient	1	

IF NATIONAL HEALTH SERVICE (A)

(a) Can I check, did you have an amenity bed which you paid for while you were in hospital or not?

Yes, had amenity bed	2
No amenity bed	3

8 How long were you in hospital on that occasion?

[*NIGHTS*]

Overnight	1
2 nights	2
3-5 nights	3
6-7 nights	4
8-14 nights	5
15-21 nights	6
over 3 weeks (specify to nearest week) _____	7

9. Did you have a bed booked to go into hospital or were you admitted as an emergency without any prior arrangements being made?

Had a bed booked	1
Admitted as emergency	2

10. Had you been into ...hosp... before as an inpatient about ..... cond. A/that pregnancy ... or was this the first time?

Had been in before	1	
First time: *emergency or maternity case*	2	onto Q23
First time: *others*	3	onto Q14

200

11. So when was the first time you went into
    ...hosp... about ....?

Before 1975 .	1	onto Q23
1975	2	
1976	3	
1977	4	

12. How long were you in hospital on that
    first occasion?

[*nights*]

overnight ...	1
2 nights	2
3-5 nights ..	3
6-7 nights ..	4
8-14 nights .	5
15-21 nights	6
over 3 weeks (specify to nearest week) _____	7

13. On that first occasion did you have a bed booked
    to go into hospital or were you admitted as an
    emergency without any prior arrangements being
    made?

Had a bed booked	1	
Admitted as emergency	2	onto Q23

14. Who arranged for you to go into ...hosp...
    on that (first) occasion?

PROMPT AS
NECESSARY

GP, family doctor	1
Private consultant or specialist	2
Outpatient dept at this hospital	3
Outpatient dept at another hospital ...	4
Other (specify)	5

201

15. How long was it altogether from when you were first
    told that you would have to go into hospital until
    you were actually admitted on that (first) occasion?

    ⌈Interviewer: note time waited⌉
    ⌊then code   ⌋

Less than a week	1
1 week - less than 2 weeks	2
2 weeks - less than 1 month ...	3
1 month - less than 3 months ..	4
3 months - less than 6 months .	5
6 months or longer (specify) ..	6

16. Had you been given any idea of how long you
    would have to wait for a bed, or not?

Yes, given some idea ...	A	ask (a)
No, not given any idea .	1	onto Q18

    IF YES, GIVEN SOME IDEA (A)

    (a) Did you actually have to wait ...

	longer than you expected	1	
RUNNING	were you admitted sooner than you expected	2	
PROMPT	or were you admitted more or less on time?	3	

17. Did you ask at anytime if you could delay going
    in until it was more convenient for you?

Yes ...	A	ask (a)
No	1	onto Q19

    IF YES (A)

    (a) Was this agreed to or not?

Yes agreed to	2	ask (i)
No, not agreed to	3	onto Q19

    IF YES AGREED TO (3)

    (i) Did they put back your admission to about the
        time you wanted, or do you think you had to
        wait much longer for a bed because you asked
        for a delay?

Put back to about time inf. wanted	1	onto Q19
Waited much longer	2	

18. Was it inconvenient not being given any idea of how
    long you might have to wait for a bed or didn't it
    really matter?

                              Yes, inconvenient   1

                              No, didn't really matter   2

19. You said you actually waited ...[see Q15 opposite]...,
    before you were admitted to hospital, did the wait
    cause you any distress or inconvenience?

                                        Yes ...   1   ask (a)

                                        No   2

    IF YES (1)

    (a) In what way was it distressing or
        inconvenient?

        0

20. Thinking now of when you actually heard that
    the hospital had a bed ready for you, how
    much notice were you given?

        DNA: Bed already booked - didn't hear from hospital ..   0   onto Q22

                          Less than 24 hours   1

                          24 hours - less than 48 hours   2

                          2 days - less than 1 week   3

                          1 week - less than 2 weeks ...   4   onto Q22

                          2 weeks or longer   5

21. Was this enough time for you or not?

                                Yes enough time ..   1

                                Not enough time ..   2

22. Can I check, were you ever given any other date for
    admission which was then postponed?

                                          Yes ..   A   ask (a)
                                          No ...   1

    IF YES (A)

    (a) Was this because you had to ask for
        the date to be changed, or had the hospital
        changed the date themselves?

                           Informant changed date .   2
                           Hospital changed date ..   3

23. APPLIES ONLY TO THOSE WITH MORE THAN ONE INPATIENT SPELL IN REFERENCE PERIOD
    (If only one inpatient spell in period go onto page 12)

    Apart from when you were in ...hosp... in _____ 197_,
    I believe you were also in hospital in ... [give dates]...
    was this also in connection with your ..cond. A...,
    or was this for something else?

         Interviewer to code (a) and (b)

    (a) Total number of inpatient spells in period,
        for condition A ──────────────────────────────▶

    (b) All other spells in period for condition A   1   onto page 12
        Some/all other spells for other conditions   2

204

24. What were your other spells in hospital for?

    ⌈ Give full details
      of condition, symptoms
      and treatment ⌋

                                    Maternity (normal delivery).   1

       Condition

       # B

                                    Maternity (normal delivery).   1

       Condition

       # C

25. *Interviewer to code:*

    No. of inpatient spells in period for condition B ⟶ ☐

    No. of inpatient spells in period for condition C ⟶ ☐

Qs26-32 are asked about <u>*one other condition only*</u>.

If <u>*only one other condition*</u> *(condition B) ask about that.*

If <u>*more than one other condition*</u> *(conditions B, C, etc), take*

condition with greatest no. of spells after <u>*excluding*</u>

maternity cases.

Interviewer to specify: which condition qns refer to (B, C) →

: no. of spells for that condition in period

26. You said you were in hospital for your ....,
in _____ 197 , (and in _____, 197 . Thinking
about the first of these spells)...

How long were you in hospital on that occasion?

[*Nights*]

overnight	1
2 nights	2
3-5 nights	3
6-7 nights	4
8-14 nights	5
15 -21 nights	6
over 3 weeks (specify to near-est week) _____	7

27. And what was the name of the hospital you were in?

specify:_____

28. Were you in hospital as a National Health Service
patient or as a private patient?

National Health Service	1
Private patient	2

29. On that (first) occasion did you have a bed
booked to go into hospital or were you admitted
as an emergency without any prior arrangements
being made?

Had a bed booked	1
Admitted as emergency	2

30. Had you been into ...hosp... before as an
inpatient about ....cond/that pregnancy ...
or was this the first time?

Had been before.	1
First time:*emergency or maternity case* ..	2
First time:*others*	3

onto page 12

206

31. Who arranged for you to go into ...hosp... on
    that occasion?

	GP, family doctor	1
	Private consultant or specialist	2
PROMPT	Outpatient dept at this hospital	3
AS	Outpatient dept at another hospital	4
NECESSARY	Other (specify)	5

32. How long altogether was it from when you were first told
    that you would have to go into hospital until you were
    actually admitted?

Less than a week	1
1 week - less than 2 weeks ...	2
2 weeks - less than 1 month ..	3
1 month - less than 3 months .	4
3 months - less than 6 months	5
6 months or longer .... (specify) _____	6

REST OF SCHEDULE REFERS ONLY TO FIRST SPELL IN HOSPITAL IN REFERENCE PERIOD Introduce and explain that all Q's now refer to that spell in hospital (for condition A) Interviewer to code from Q9 p4. For first spell in hospital in ref. period informant		
had a bed booked	1	ask Q33
was an emergency	2	onto Q42

TRANSPORT TO THE HOSPITAL

33. How long did it take you to get to the hospital?

About 15 (1–22) mins	1	
About 30 (23–37) mins	2	
About 45 (38–50) mins	3	
About 1 hour or longer (51 mins or more) specify: ———————————	4	
SPONTANEOUS: Don't know	0	

34. How did you get to the hospital, did the hospital send an ambulance or hospital car for you, or did you make your own way there?

Hospital sent ambulance/car	1	onto Q36
Made own way there	2	

35. Would you have preferred the hospital to have laid on transport to get you there, or wasn't it really necessary?

Would have preferred hospital transport	1	ask (a)
Not really necessary	2	onto p.17

IF WOULD HAVE PREFERRED HOSPITAL TRANSPORT(1)

(a) Why would you have preferred the hospital to have laid on transport to get you there?

0

onto p.17

36. What sort of transport did the hospital send for you?

PROMPT AS NECESSARY	Ambulance - lying down or stretcher ..	1
	Ambulance - sitting or wheelchair	2
	a hospital car	3

37. Were you given a specific time when the ambulance/car would pick you up?

	Yes ...	1
	No	A	ask (a)

IF NO (A)

(a) Did you find this inconvenient or didn't it really matter that much?

Yes it was inconvenient .	2	
No, didn't really matter	3	onto Q41

38. Did the ambulance/car come at about the time it was supposed to?

Yes ...	1	onto Q41
No	2	

39. Was it early or was it late?

Early	1	ask (a)
Late	2	ask (b)

IF EARLY (1)

(a) About how early did it come?

Specify no. of minutes ⟶

IF LATE (2)

(b) About how late did it come?

Specify no. of minutes ⟶

209

40. Did it matter to you that it failed to come at
    about the right time, or didn't it really matter
    that much?

                              Yes, it mattered   1
                              No, didn't really matter ..   2

41. And bearing in mind your condition was your journey
    to hospital reasonably comfortable?

                                        Yes ...   1   onto p.17
                                        No   2   ask (a)

    IF NO (2)

    (a) What could have been done to have made your
        journey to hospital in the ambulance/car
        more comfortable?

                              Nothing   1
                              Don't know   2   onto p.17
                              Other (specify)   3

                                   Onto p.17

42. TO ALL EMERGENCY ADMISSIONS

    How did you get to the hospital, did you go by
    ambulance, did you make your own way there or
    what?

                              Ambulance   1
                              Made own way there   2   onto Q46
                              Other (specify) ..   3

43. What sort of ambulance did the hospital send
    for you, was it a stretcher ambulance, or one
    you could sit up in?

                    Ambulance - lying down or stretcher   1
                    Ambulance - sitting up or wheelchair ...   2
       SPONTANEOUS :   Hospital car   3

210

44. How long did it take for the ambulance/car to come?

Don't know - was unconscious, had no awareness of time 1

Can't remember 2

Less than 15 mins 3

Other: specify no of minutes ⌐

└→ ☐☐☐ ask (a)

IF WAITED 15 MINS OR MORE

(a) Do you think the ambulance/car took an unreasonable length of time to come or not?

Yes ... 1

No 2

45. Bearing in mind your condition was your journey to hospital reasonably comfortable?

Don't know - unconscious ... 1 ⌐
Yes 2   } onto Q47
No .... 3 └ - ask (a)

IF NO (3)

(a) What could have been done to have made your journey to hospital in the ambulance more comfortable?

0

Nothing ...... 1 ⌐
Don't know ... 2   } onto Q47
Other (specify) 3 └

┌──────────┐
│ onto Q47 │
└──────────┘

46. Would you have preferred the hospital to have sent an ambulance for you, or wasn't it necessary?

Would have preferred ambulance 1   ask (a)

Not necessary 2

IF WOULD HAVE PREFERRED AMBULANCE (1)

(a) Why would you have preferred the hospital to have sent an ambulance for you?

0

47. How long did it take you to get to the hospital?

Don't know - was unconscious, had no awareness of time	0	
Can't remember	9	
About 15 (1-22) mins	1	
About 30 (23-37) mins	2	
About 45 (38-50) mins	3	
About 1 hour or longer (51 mins or more) specify:_____	4	

48. And after you got to the hospital how long was it before you were seen by a doctor?

Unconscious dazed-don't know ...	0	
About 5 or 10 (1-12) minutes (incl. immediately)	1	onto p.17
About 15 (13-22) minutes	2	
About 30 (23-37) minutes	3	
About 45 (38-50) minutes	4	
About 1 hour or longer (51 minutes or more) specify _____	5	

49. Were you told why you had to wait to be seen?

Yes told	1
No not told .	2

50. Do you personally think this was an unreasonable time to wait or not?

Yes, unreasonable	1	ask (a)
No, not unreasonable ..	2	

IF YES UNREASONABLE (1)

(a) Why is that?

Q's 51-60 (WHITE PAGES) APPLY TO CHILD PATIENTS AGED UNDER 14
ONLY
(Others go onto Q61)

Ask proxy

51. When (..child...) was in hospital was he/she in
    a children's ward or in a ward with adults?

Children's/baby's ward	1
Ward with adults	2

52. Would you have preferred (..child...) to have been
    in a children's ward, would you have preferred
    him/her to be with adults or didn't you think it
    mattered that much?

Preferred children's ward .	1	ask Q53(a)
Preferred with adults	2	ask Q53(b)
Didn't matter that much ...	3	onto Q54

53. Why [would you have preferred / did you prefer] him/her to be in a ....

    (a) children's ward?

    ∩

    (b) ward with adults?

    ∩

54. I shall be asking you about ...child... treatment
    later, but thinking about the ward he/she was in,
    was there anything about the <u>facilities</u> or the <u>condition</u>
    of the ward that you were dissatisfied with?

Yes, dissatisfied ...	1	ask (a)
No, satisfied	2	

IF YES DISSATISFIED (<u>1</u>)

(a) What were you dissatisfied with?

0

55. When ...child... was in hospital were you asked if
    you would like to stay overnight or even longer so
    that you would be near him/her?

Yes, asked	1	
No, not asked	A	ask (a)

IF NO NOT ASKED (A)

(a) Would you have wanted to stay at the
    hospital, or wasn't it really necessary?

Wanted to stay	2	on to Q.59
Not really necessary	3	

56. Did you actually stay at the hospital overnight or not?

Yes, stayed	1
No, didn't stay	2

57. What arrangements did the hospital make for you to
    stay there?

---

58. And were the arrangments for your staying there
    satisfactory or not?

                                    Yes, satisfactory ...   1
                                    Not satisfactory   2   ask(a)

    IF NOT SATISFACTORY (2)

    (a) What were you dissatisfied with?

    ()

215

59. If you wanted to find out how ...child... was,
was the hospital happy for you to phone up at
any time, or did you get the impression they
didn't really like it?

	Hospital was happy about phoning ...	1
	Didn't really like it	2
SPONTANEOUS:	Can't say, don't know	3

60. Some hospitals nowadays encourage parents to spend
quite long periods at the hospital, helping out
and keeping their own and other children amused ...
Do you personally think this is a good idea or not?

Yes a good idea ...	1	on to Q113 p.36
Not a good idea ...	2	ask (a)

IF NOT A GOOD IDEA (2)

(a) Why don't you think it's a particularly
good idea?

on to Q113 p.36

216

THE WARD AND ITS FACILITIES (Applies only to patients aged 14 and over)

61. While you were in hospital on that occasion, were you
    in a room on your own for all or part of your stay,
    or were you always in with other patients?

In a room on own - all of the time	1	onto Q66
In a room on own - part of the time ...	2	
Always with other patients	3	

62. (When you were in with other patients)
    Apart from curtains was the ward or room you were in
    divided or partitioned into sections or bays in any way?

Yes, divided up	1
Not divided up	2

63. How many beds were there in your ward/part of
    the ward?

up to 4	1
5-10	2
11-15	3
16-25	4
More than 25	5

64. For most of the time you were there ...

RUNNING	were all or nearly all of the beds occupied .	1
PROMPT	were only about half occupied	2
	or were less than half of them occupied?.....	3

217

65. Thinking about the number of beds in your (part of
the) ward do you personally think there were ...

RUNNING PROMPT	too few beds	1	ask (a)
	too many beds	2	ask (b)
	or were there about the right number? .	3	

IF TOO FEW BEDS (1)

(a) What makes you say that there were
too few beds?

∩

IF TOO MANY BEDS (2)

(b) What makes you say that there were
too many beds?

∩

66. Were patients allowed to smoke in the room/ward
you were in, or did they have to go somewhere
else for a smoke?

Could smoke in room/ward	1	ask (a)
Had to go elsewhere	2	ask (b)
Patients not allowed to smoke anywhere in hospital ...	3	
Don't know	4	

IF COULD SMOKE IN ROOM (1)

(a) How did you feel about patients being
allowed to smoke in your room/ward?

Pleased – in favour	1
Didn't mind	2
Objected – against	3

IF HAD TO GO ELSEWHERE (2) or NOT ALLOWED (3)

(b) How did you feel about patients not
being allowed to smoke (in your room/ward)?

Pleased – in favour	1
Didn't mind	2
Objected – against	3

CHECK

67. Do you smoke at all yourself?

Yes	1
No	2

68. Was there a dayroom or rest room where you could go to sit when you were out of bed?

Yes	1	
No	A	ask (a)
Don't know .	2	

IF NO (A)

(a) Would you have liked to have been able to go and sit somewhere else when you were out of bed, or weren't you really bothered?

Would have liked dayroom ..	3
Not really bothered	4
Bedfast	5

69. Thinking now about the facilities for patients ... Was there a TV you could watch while you were in hospital?

Yes	1	ask (a)
No	2	
Don't know .	3	

IF YES (1)

(a) Was it in the room/ward you were in, or did you have to go somewhere else if you wanted to watch it?

CODE ALL THAT APPLY

In same ward patient was in	1	ask (i)
In patient's own single room	2	
Somewhere else	3	

IF IN SAME WARD (1)

(i) Did it disturb you at all when it was on or not?

Yes, (sometimes) ...	1
No	2

219

70. While you were in hospital did you have ....

    INDIV. PROMPT   a hospital radio, or earphones?......   1
    CODE FIRST
    THAT APPLIES   did you take your own radio with you?   2   onto Q73

                                neither of these ....   A   ask (a)

IF CODED (A)

(a) Would you have liked to have been
    able to listen to the radio in bed, or
    weren't you really bothered?

                     Yes would have liked radio ...   3
                                         onto Q73
                     No, not bothered   4

71. Did the hospital radio (and earphones) work
all right or didn't you use them?

                     Yes, worked all right   1
                     No, didn't work properly   2
                     Not used   3   onto Q73

72. And were you generally able to get the
stations you wanted to listen to on the
hospital radio or not?

                                    Yes ...   1
                                    No   2

73. Was there a telephone that patients could use to make telephone calls out?

Yes	1	
No	A	ask (a)

IF NO (A)

(a) Would you have liked to have been able to make telephone calls out or weren't you really bothered?

Yes would have liked a phone.	2	onto Q75
No, not really bothered	3	

74. Could patients also take incoming telephone calls?

Yes ...	A	ask (a)
No	1	

IF YES (A)

(a) How did you personally feel about patients being able to take incoming calls?

In favour, pleased it was possible	2
Didn't mind ....,.	3
Against, objected to it	4

75. Most hospitals have their own shop, or run a ward service where patients can buy newspapers, magazines, sweets or cigarettes, toilet articles and so on ... Was there anything like that in the hospital you were in?

CODE ALL THAT
APPLY

Yes a hospital shop	1
Yes a ward service	2
No, neither	3

[If both a hospital shop (1) and a ward service (2) go onto Q77]
(Others ask Q76)

76. Would you have found a hospital shop/(or) a ward service useful, or weren't you really bothered?

Yes useful	1
No, not really bothered	2

221

77. Can we go on now to talk about the food you
    had while you were in hospital ...

    Were you on a special diet at all while you
    were there?

    PROMPT AS   Yes, all the time ...   1
    NECESSARY   Yes, some of the time   2
                       No   3

78. And could you choose what you wanted to eat
    from a menu, or was there never any choice?

                              Choice   1
                              No choice ..   2

79. Some people have told us that they felt that
    the meals were served at unsuitable times in
    hospital ...
    How did you personally feel about the times
    that the meals were served while you were in
    hospital?

        0

80. And were you generally satisfied or dissatisfied
    with the food?

                         Satisfied   1
                         Dissatisfied ..   2   ask (a)

    IF DISSATISFIED (2)

    (a) What was unsatisfactory about the food?

        0

222

81. Now about your hospital bed ... it's sometimes difficult to get used to a strange bed but was your hospital bed as comfortable as it could be bearing in mind your condition?

Yes	1	
No	2	ask (a)

IF NO (2)

(a) What was the trouble?

0

82. What time were you usually woken up in the morning?

	5.00 am - 5.30	1
	5.31 am - 6.00	2
PROMPT AS NECESSARY	6.01 am - 6.30	3
	6.31 am - 7.00	4
[If range given code mid-point]	7.01 am - 7.30	5
	7.31 am - 8.00	6
	After 8.00 am	7

83. Did you personally think this was ...

	too early	1
RUNNING PROMPT	too late	2
	or about right?.	3

84. During the daytime were you generally disturbed by the amount of noise or not?

Yes ...	1
No	2

85. If you wanted to rest during the daytime could you
usually manage to do so?

Yes	1	
No	2	ask (a)
Don't know, didn't want to rest	3	

IF NO (2)

(a) Was that because of the noise or
for some other reason?

Because of noise	1
Other reason (specify) .	2

86. At night were you generally disturbed by noise and
things going on or not?

Yes, disturbed	A	ask (a)(b)
Not disturbed	1	

IF YES,DISTURBED (A)

(a) Did the noise and things going on
make it difficult for you to get a
fair night's sleep, or wasn't it that bad?

Made it difficult to sleep	2
Not that bad	3

(b) Who or what was it that disturbed
you?

0

87. I've asked you about the times that meals were
served in hospital and about what time you were
woken up in the mornings. I'd now like to talk
about all the routine things that happen each day
while you're in hospital, for example doctors
rounds, visiting times and so on ...

When you were first admitted to hospital did any
of the nurses or other staff explain the daily
routine to you?

Yes, was explained .	1
No, not explained ..	2

224

88. Do you think from your own experience as a patient
    that being told about the daily routine quite
    soon after admission is ...

RUNNING PROMPT	Very important	1
	important	2
	or not important? ...	3

89. What about the washing and bathing facilities
    you had in hospital ... were they satisfactory
    or not?

Yes washing and bathing facilities satisfactory	1	
No, not satisfactory	2	ask (a)
Don't know, not used	3	onto Q91

IF NO, NOT SATISFACTORY (2)

(a) What was unsatisfactory?

0

Not enough washbasins ..	1
Not enough baths	2
Other (specify)	3

90. And did you personally have enough privacy when you
    were washing and bathing?

Yes, enough privacy when washing and bathing ..	1	
No	A	ask (a)

IF NO (A)

(a) Did this bother you ...

RUNNING PROMPT	quite a lot	2
	only a little	3
	or didn't it really bother you at all?.	4

91. How about the W.C.'s, were you satisfied with the
toilet facilities or not?

Yes, satisfied	1	
Not satisfied	2	ask (a)
Don't know, not used .	3	

IF NOT SATISFIED (2)

(a) What was unsatisfactory about the
toilet facilities?

Not enough toilets ...	1
Other (specify)	2

0

92. While you were in hospital, did you ever have
to have a bedpan (or bottle - MEN) because you
were unable to get out of bed?

Yes	1	
No	2	onto Q95
Had catheter - no bedpan/bottle	3	

93. Were there ever any difficulties in getting a
bedpan or bottle when you wanted one?

Yes.....	1
No	2

94. Was it always taken away promptly after use?

Yes, always prompt	1
Prompt during day, but not at night	2
No, never prompt	3

TO ALL

95. Apart from the toilets and the washing and bathing
facilities were you satisfied with the cleanliness
of the room/ward you were in?

Yes	1	
No	2	
DNA blind	3	onto Q97

96. And were you satisfied with the general
    condition of the room/ward you were in
    - its decoration, layout, tidiness and
    so on?

Yes, satisfied ...	1	
No, dissatisfied	2	ask (a)

IF NO DISSATISFIED (2)

(a) What in particular were you dissatisfied
    with?

0

97. Did you generally find that your hospital room/ward
    was kept at ....

	about the right temperature	1	
RUNNING	that it was generally kept too warm	2	
PROMPT	or that it was generally not kept warm enough for you ?.......	3	

98. Thinking back to your own experience as a patient in hospital, if you had to go into hospital again would you prefer to be ...

	in a room on your own	1	
RUNNING PROMPT	in a small ward with up to about six beds	2	on to Q.100
	or in a ward with more than about six beds?	3	on to Q.101

99. Why would you prefer to be in a room on your own rather than with other patients?

0

on to Q.102

100. Why would you prefer to be in a small ward with up to six beds rather than be on your own or in a larger ward?

0

on to Q.102

101. Why would you prefer to be in a bigger ward rather than be in a room on your own, or in a small ward?

0

VISITING ARRANGEMENTS (Patients aged 14 and over only)

We would like to find out what you thought about the
visiting arrangements while you were in hospital ...

102. Were visitors allowed every day, including
Saturdays and Sundays, or only on some days?

Every day incl. Sat and Sun	1	
Only on some days	2	ask (a)
Don't know	3	

IF ONLY ON SOME DAYS (2)

(a) On how many days were visitors allowed?

specify number ⟶

103. (On the days that visiting was allowed)
Was there visiting ....

	every afternoon	1
RUNNING	on only some afternoons	2
PROMPT	or was there no afternoon visiting at all?	3
SPONTANEOUS:	Don't know...............	4

104. And (on the days that visiting was allowed) was there
visiting ...

	every evening	1
RUNNING	only on some evenings	2
PROMPT	or was there no evening visiting at all?	3
SPONTANEOUS:	Don't know............................	4

CHECK IF THERE WAS VISITING EVERY AFTERNOON AND
EVERY EVENING (Q103 AND Q104 coded 1) GO ON TO
Q106

Others ask Q105

105. Would you personally have liked afternoon and evening
visiting every day (that visitors were allowed) or not?

Yes would have liked that ...	1
No	2

106. On the whole were the visiting hours convenient
for your visitors or not?

Yes, convenient ...	1
Not convenient	2	ask (a)
No visitors	3

IF NOT CONVENIENT (2)

(a) Why were the hours not convenient for
your visitors?

0

---

107. Thinking about all the visitors to the ward, not just
your own visitors ...

As a patient, would you have preferred ...

	longer visiting hours	1
RUNNING	shorter visiting hours	2
PROMPT	or were you quite satisfied with the visiting hours?	3

---

108. In practice, was there a limit on the number of
visitors you were allowed to have?

PROMPT AS	Yes, limit at all sessions ..	1	ask (a)(b)
NECESSARY	Yes, limit at some sessions .	2
	No limit	3

IF YES, AT ALL SESSIONS (1)

(a) What was the limit?

specify ⟶ [|]

(b) Do you personally think this was ...

RUNNING	too many	1
PROMPT	too few	2	on to Q110
	or about the right number? .	3

109. Do you think they should have (always) put a
limit on the number of visitors allowed or not?

                        Yes, should have limited nos. ...   1

                        No   2

110. Were children allowed to visit in the room/ward
you were in?

                        Yes at any session   1

                        Yes but only at some sessions ...   2

                        No not at all .... , 3

                        Don't know   4

111. How do you personally feel about children visiting
people in hospital?

    []

112. And the last question about visiting ... did
you personally have enough privacy when you
had visitors?

                        Yes   1

                        No ....   A   ask (a)

                        No visitors ...   2

    IF NO (A)

    (a) Did this bother you ...

                        quite a lot   3

        RUNNING   only a little   4

        PROMPT   or didn't it really bother
                        you at all?   5

231

TREATMENT ⎡ Qs 113 - 115 refer to items of treatment A-H as
⎢ specified in grid below, and answers to these
⎣ questions are coded in the grid. ⎤

Introduce: Can we talk now about various sorts of treatment
that you might have had while you were in hospital.

113. While you were in hospital on that occasion ....

Did you have .... INDIVIDUALLY PROMPT ITEMS A-H
AND CODE BELOW Yes = 1
No = 2

		Q113	
		YES	NO
A	a blood sample taken or a blood test?	,, 1	2...
B	any injections?	,, 1	2...
C	X-rays?	,, 1	2...
D	physiotherapy?	,, 1	2...
E	give a water or urine specimen?..........................	,, 1	2...
F	a general anaesthetic - (being put to sleep for a short while)?...	,, 1	2...
G	stitches or clips or have them removed?	,, 1	2...
H	dressings done, changed or removed?	,, 1	2...

⎡ Ask Q114 for each item coded Yes (1) except G & H
⎣ if Q114 DNA see instruction above Q115 ⎤

114 Thinking about when you had (... the blood sample taken ...)
were you told enough about why it was necessary?

RING CODES IN GRID   Yes, told enough   = 3

No, not told enough = 4

For each item coded (4) - NO, NOT TOLD ENOUGH ask (a)

(a) Were you bothered by this or not?

RING CODES IN GRID   Yes, bothered   = 5

No, not bothered = 6

If <u>any</u> item coded Yes (1) at Q113 ask Q115
if <u>no</u> item coded Yes (1) go to next page

115. You said you had ..... [read out items of treatment
received] were any of these things particularly
unpleasant or not?

EITHER CODE HERE: none of the treatment was unpleasant ...   0

OR RING CODE 7 BELOW for each item of treatment that
was unpleasant

For each item coded (7) - UNPLEASANT ask (a)

(a) Could anything have been done to make it less
unpleasant?

RING CODES BELOW: Yes, something could be done = 8

                             No, nothing could be done = 9

Q114		Q114 (a)		Q115	Q115(a)	
YES - told enough	N O - not told enough	YES bothered	NO - not bothered	UN-PLEASANT	YES	NO
3 .... 4		..... 5 ....,6		,.,.. 7,,,,,,	,...,8 ....,9	
3 ..'.................. 4		..... 5 ....,6		,.,.. 7	....,8 ....,9	
3 .... 4		..... 5 ..,.....,6 ,,...		,.,.. 7	....,8 ....,9	
3 .... 4		..... 5 ....,6 ,,...		,.,.. 7	....,8 .....,9	
3 .... 4		..... 5 ....,6		,.,..,7,,,,,	....,8 9	
3 ...·············· 4		..... 5 .... 6		.....7	....,8 9	
				..... 7	.....,8 9	
				..... 7	.....,8 9	

REMEMBER Q115 IS ABOVE GRID

233

Qs 116-121 APPLY ONLY TO PATIENTS AGED 14 AND OVER
(child patients under 14 go onto Q122)

116. Some people have told us that one of the things they
dislike about being in hospital is the lack of
privacy ...

Did you personally feel that you always had
enough privacy when you were being examined
or treated?

Yes, always	1	onto Q121
No	2	

117. When you were being examined or treated
could other patients overhear what was
being said to you or not?

Yes, other patients could hear	1	ask (a)(b)
No, other patients could not hear .	2	
Don't know	3	

IF YES (1)

(a) Did this bother you ...

quite a lot ....,........	1	
RUNNING PROMPT only a little	2	
or didn't it really bother you at all? .....,....................,.........	3	

(b) Did it ever bother you overhearing what
was being said to other patients?

Yes ..	1	
No ...	2	
Couldn't hear/no other patients	3	

234

118. And when you were being examined or treated could
you be seen by other patients or not?

Yes, could be seen	1	ask (a)(b)
No, could not be seen ...	2	
Don't know	3	

IF YES (1)

(a) Did this bother you ...

	quite a lot ..,...............	1
RUNNING PROMPT	only a little	2
	or didn't it really bother you at all?	3

(b) Did it ever bother you seeing other
patients being treated or not?

Yes ...	1
No	2
Couldn't see/no other patients .	3

119. Were there ever any medical students present
while you were being examined or treated?

Yes ...	1	
No	2	onto Q121

120. Were you asked if you agreed to their being
present or not?

Yes (incl. sometimes) .	1	
No, never	A	ask (a)(b)
Can't remember	2	

IF NO, NEVER (A)

(a) Did you mind not being asked, or
weren't you really bothered?

Yes, minded	3
Not really bothered ...	4

(b) And did you mind the medical students
being there, or didn't it really worry
you?

Yes, minded	1
No, not worried .	2

235

121. Did any of the doctors discuss your condition
     or treatment with other people as if you
     weren't there?

                                        Yes   1   ask (a)
                                        No   2

IF YES (1)

(a) How did you feel about this?

     0

TO ALL

122. Most people are a bit apprehensive about what's
     going to happen to them in hospital ...
     On the whole do you think that the doctors and
     nurses did all they could to set your mind at
     rest about what was going to happen while you
     were in hospital?

                                        Yes   1
                                        No   2

123. While you were in hospital do you think you were
     always told enough about how you (and the baby)
     were progressing?

                    Yes, always told enough   1   .onto Q126
                    Wanted to know more ...   2

124. Did you feel that you could ask the doctors to
     tell you what you wanted to know, or not?

                         Yes could ask all doctors   1
         PROMPT AS   Yes could only ask some   ask (a)
         NECESSARY   doctors, not others   2
                         No, could not ask any
                         doctors   3   ask Q125

IF YES COULD ASK ALL OR SOME DOCTORS (1) or (2)

(a) When you asked the doctors what you wanted to know,
    did you generally get a satisfactory answer?

                         Yes   1
                         No   2   onto Q126
                         Never asked any questions   3

236

125. Why did you feel that you couldn't ask the doctors
what you wanted to know?

0

Don't know/just didn't ask	1
Other (specify)	2

126. Did you always understand what the doctors told
you about your condition and treatment, or would
you sometimes have liked it explained in everyday
language?

Understood	1	
Would have liked it explained .	A	ask (a)

IF WOULD LIKE IT EXPLAINED (A)

(a) Did you ever ask any other doctor or nurse at
the hospital to explain what had been said to you?

Yes	2
No	3

127. Apart from using medical terms, did you ever
have any difficulty in simply understanding
what any of the doctors were saying?

Yes, had difficulty .	1	ask (a)
No, no difficulty ...	2	

IF YES HAD DIFFICULTY (1)

(a) What was the difficulty?

0

CHECK: if informant didn't understand what doctor said
either at Q126 (coded A) or at Q127 (coded 1) ask Q128
(Others go onto Q120)

128. How did you personally feel about not always
understanding what the doctors were saying?
Were you ...

	Not really bothered ...	1
RUNNING	Worried or upset by it	2
PROMPT	or were you embarrassed? .	3

129. I'd now like to ask you briefly about how you felt
about the staff you met while you were in hospital.
Thinking about the nurses you met while you were
in hospital,did you find that...

RUNNING PROMPT	all of them were considerate	1
	that most of them were considerate	2
	or that only a few of them were considerate?	3
SPONTANEOUS:	not met enough/any - can't say	4

130. And how about medical staff, people like
physiotherapists, radiographers and dieticians,
did you find that ...

RUNNING PROMPT	all of them were nice to you	1
	that most of them were nice to you	2
	or that only a few of them were nice to you?	3
SPONTANEOUS:	not met enough/any - can't say	4

131. And how about the non-medical staff at the
hospital - the porters, receptionists and
orderlies; were ...

RUNNING PROMPT	all of them helpful	1
	most of them helpful	2
	or only a few of them helpful?	3
SPONTANEOUS:	not met enough/any - can't say	4

TO PATIENTS AGED UNDER 14
(Others go onto Q133)
Ask Proxy

132 Do you think the doctors and nurses did all they
could to reassure and comfort your child, or do
you think they could perhaps have done more?

they did all they could	1	
Could have done more	2	ask(a)

IF COULD HAVE DONE MORE (2)

(a) What in particular do you think they could
have done?

Ω

133. Although I've talked about the doctors and nurses at the hospital I haven't mentioned hospital almoners or social workers; they help and advise patients who might be worried about their home, their family or their job while they are in hospital ...

Did an almoner or hospital social worker visit you after you were admitted to hospital or not?

Yes, social worker visited	1	
No visit by social worker	A	ask (a)

IF NO VISIT BY SOCIAL WORKER (A)

(a) Did you have any worries or problems that you would have liked to talk over with a social worker?

Yes	2
No	3

134. And of all the people you came into contact with while you were there - doctors, nurses, ward staff, other patients, anyone at all, who did most to help you adapt to being in hospital?

	Nursing sister	1
	Auxiliary nurses	2
CODE ONE	Other nurses	3
ONLY	Hospital doctors	4
	Own GP/family doctor	5
	Relatives	6
	Other patients	7
	Other (specify)	8

135. And on the whole do you feel you were treated as an individual or did you feel that you were just another case?

Individual	1
Just another case ..	2

239

DISCHARGE
I'd now like to ask you about the arrangements made for
discharging you from hospital ...

136. When you were told that you were being discharged, was
there enough time for you to make any arrangements that
you had to?

Yes enough time	1
Not enough time	2

137. How did you get home, did you go by ambulance
or hospital car, or did you make your own
arrangements?

Went by ambulance/hospital car	1	
Made own arrangements	A	ask (a)

IF MADE OWN ARRANGEMENTS (A)

(a) Would you have preferred it if you had gone
home by ambulance or hospital car or wasn't
it really necessary?

Preferred hospital transport ..	2	ask (i)
Not really necessary	3	

IF PREFERRED HOSPITAL TRANSPORT (2)

(i) Why would you have preferred to have
gone home by hospital transport?

()

138. And before you were discharged from hospital did you
have any worries or doubts about how you would be able
to manage once you were home?

Yes, had worries ...	A	ask (a)
No worries	1	onto Q140

IF YES HAD WORRIES (A)

(a) Did anyone like the almoner or social worker
come and talk to you about this?

Yes	2	onto Q139
No one seen	3	ask (i)

IF NO ONE SEEN (3)

(i) Would you have liked to have talked it
over with someone, or weren't you
that worried?

Would have liked to have talked to someone	1	onto Q140
Not that worried	2	

240

139. Were they able to make any arrangements for you to
be helped once you were home?

Yes   1   ask (a)

No   2

IF YES (1)

(a) What did they do?

140. Once you got home were you able to manage all right,
or should the hospital have arranged (more) help
for you?

Managed all right   1

Should have arranged help ..   2

141. In general is there anything (more) that the hospital
could have done to help you once you were at home?

Yes   1   ask (a)

No   2

IF YES (1)

(a) What (else) could have been done to help you
once you were home?

0

142. On the whole were you ...

quite happy to leave hospital when
you did   1

RUNNING   do you think you should have been
PROMPT   discharged sooner   2

or do you think you should have
stayed in longer?................   3

143. After you were discharged from hospital how long
     was it before you saw your GP/family doctor?

Not yet seen GP	0	onto Q145
less than 3 days	1	
3 days - less than 1 week ...	2	
1 week - less than 2 weeks ..	3	
2 weeks - less than 1 month .	4	
1 month or longer (specify) _____	5	
SPONTANEOUS: Can't remember	9	

144. The first time you saw him after you were discharged
     had he already heard from the hospital about how you
     had got on or not?

Yes, had heard	1	onto Q146
No, had not heard ...	2	
Don't know, not sure	3	

145. Did the hospital give you a letter or a note to
     take to your GP the next time you saw him?

Yes, given a note/letter ...	1
No note or letter	2

146. After you left hospital, did you have to go back
     to hospital as an outpatient at all?

Yes	A	ask (a)
No	1	

IF YES (A)

(a) Are you still going back as an outpatient as
    a result of your stay in hospital or have you
    finished all your follow-up visits?

Still going ...	2
Finished	3

242

147. I've talked in detail about many aspects of your stay
in hospital, but before I finish I'd like to ask a
few more general questions ...

Were you ever sent or given a booklet or leaflet, which
told you about the hospital, its facilities, visiting
arrangements and so on?

	Yes	A	ask (a)(b)
IF YES (A)	No	1	

(a) Were you given it ....

RUNNING	before you were admitted .	2
PROMPT	or after you were admitted?..	3

(b) Did you find it ...

RUNNING	Very useful	1	onto Q148
PROMPT	fairly useful	2	
	or not at all useful?....	3	ask (i)

IF NOT AT ALL USEFUL (3)

(i) What makes you say that?

0

148. Were you told at anytime how to go about making a
complaint to the Hospital Authorities, should you
wish to make one?

Yes told	1
No, not told	2

149. If you had to go back into hospital again would you ...

RUNNING	definitely want to go into ...hosp...	
PROMPT	again	1
	definitely not want to go there again ...	2
	or wouldn't you mind either way?	3

150. Would you say that on the whole the hospital service
for inpatients is ...

	very good	1
RUNNING	good	2
PROMPT	has its faults	3
	or is poor?	4

CLASSIFICATION, OCCUPATION, INDUSTRY AND INCOME

(If informant is under 16 collect all information from parent)

Introduce:

151 HOUSEHOLD COMPOSITION

RELATIONSHIP TO OUTPATIENT		HOH	H' WIFE	SEX		AGE LAST BIRTH- DAY	MARITAL STATUS			WORKING STATUS			
	Office use			M	F		M	S	Wid Sep Div	FULL TIME (over 30)	PART TIME (over 10-30)	UN- EMPLOYED	NOT WORKING
PATIENT		1	2	1	2		1	2	3	1	2	3	4
		1	2	1	2		1	2	3	1	2	3	4
		1	2	1	2		1	2	3	1	2	3	4
		1	2	1	2		1	2	3	1	2	3	4
		1	2	1	2		1	2	3	1	2	3	4
		1	2	1	2		1	2	3	1	2	3	4
		1	2	1	2		1	2	3	1	2	3	4
		1	2	1	2		1	2	3	1	2	3	4
		1	2	1	2		1	2	3	1	2	3	4
		1	2	1	2		1	2	3	1	2	3	4
		1	2	1	2		1	2	3	1	2	3	4.

Number of persons in household ....

IF PATIENT IS AGED 16 OR OVER AND NOT WORKING ASK Q151(a)

151. (a) Are you ...

	retired	1
PROMPT AS NECESSARY	permanently sick/disabled	2
	temp. off-sick - no job to return to	3
	housewife	4
CODE FIRST THAT APPLIES	at school	5
	in other full-time education?	6

152. PATIENT'S OCCUPATION OR IF RETIRED LAST MAIN OCCUPATION		154. HOH'S OCCUPATION OR IF RETIRED LAST MAIN OCCUPATION	
DNA Patient aged under 16 or never worked	X onto Q154	DNA Patient is HOH	X onto Q156
What is your job? What do you actually do?		What is your (..HOH's) job? What does he actually do?	

153. PATIENT'S INDUSTRY		155. HOH'S INDUSTRY	
What does the firm/ organisation you work for actually make or do?		What does the firm/ organisation he works for actually make or do?	
Are you an employee .	1	Is he an employee .	1
or self-employed? ...	2	or self-employed? .	2
If manager,superintendent, self-employed:		If manager, superintendent, self-employed:	
How many people work in the establishment?		How many people work in the establishment?	
1-24 ..	X	1-24 ..	X
25 + ..	Y	25 + ..	Y

245

INCOME:

156. Please could you look at this card (HAND OVER INCOME
CARD) and tell me into which of the 8 groups your
own income falls. This includes the income from all
sources, after income tax, National Insurance and other
deductions have been taken off.

CODE BELOW AND THEN REPEAT QUESTION FOR HOH's INCOME

Per week	Annual	Patient	HOH
Nil	Nil	1	1
up to £10	up to £520	2	2
over £10 - £20	over £520 - £1040 ...	3	3
over £20 - £40	over £1040 - £2080 ..	4	4
over £40 - £60	over £2080 - £3120 ..	5	5
over £60 - £80	over £3120 - £4160 ..	6	6
over £80 - £100	over £4160 - £5200 ..	7	7
over £100	over £5200	8	8
If patient is HOH ring code		9	
Don't know			9
Refused/not asked - code and write in reason		0	0

CHECK: If patient AND/OR HOH is earning less than
£2080 (codes 1 - 4) ask Q157
(If both patient AND HOH are earning over £2080 go onto Q158)

157. Could I check, are you (is your ..HOH ..)
currently receiving supplementary benefit?

	Patient	HOH
Yes, is receiving supp. benefit....	1	1
No	2	2
Don't know		3
If patient is HOH ring code	3	

246

1 58. Finally apart from the things we've discussed already
is there anything else that you would like to say
about your stay in...hosp....for your.....
cond........?

                                              No   1

                                              Yes (specify)   2

⎡ THANK INFORMANT FOR CO-OPERATION ⎤
⎣ LEAVE LEAFLET   ⎦

Appendix III

Additional tables

Table 1: How long patients attending ancillary departments waited for their first appointment

How long patients waited for their first appointment:	Patient attended:	
	ancillary departments	consultative outpatients
	cum %	cum %
7 days or less	55	25
8–14 days	72	41
15–21 days	85	56
22–28 days	88	68
over 4 wks–5 wks	90	74
over 5 wks–6 wks	92	79
over 6 wks–3 months	99	93
over 3 months	100	100
Base: all who had an appointment for their outpatient visit=100%	89	532

Table 2: Proportions of patients in wards of different sizes who found the washing and bathing facilities satisfactory

Washing and bathing facilities were:	No. of beds in ward or part of ward:					All
	up to 4[1]	5–10	11–15	16–25	over 25	
	%	%	%	%	%	%
satisfactory	82	81	75	83	73	80
unsatisfactory	18	19	25	17	27	20
Base: all inpatients aged 14 and over=100%[2]	212	189	97	127	56	681

1. includes 39 patients who were in a room on their own throughout their stay in hospital
2. excludes those who did not use the washing or bathing facilities (bedfast)

Table 3: Proportions of patients in wards of different sizes who found the toilet (WC) facilities satisfactory

Toilet facilities were:	No. of beds in ward or part of ward:					All
	up to 4[1]	5–10	11–15	16–25	over 25	
	%	%	%	%	%	%
satisfactory	89	86	82	84	63	84
unsatisfactory	11	14	18	16	37	16
Base: all inpatients aged 14 and over=100%[2]	210	189	97	127	56	679

1. includes 39 patients who were in a room on their own throughout their stay in hospital
2. excludes those who did not use the toilet facilities (bedfast)

Table 4: Proportions of patients in different age groups who found the waiting area in the department they had attended very comfortable

Patients who found the waiting area:	Patients aged					All men	All women
	0–16	17–34	35–54	55–64	65 & over		
	%	%	%	%	%	%	%
very comfortable	19	17	28	35	50	26	31
all right	71	70	63	61	47	65	62
rather uncomfortable	8	11	8	2	2	7	6
very uncomfortable	2	2	1	2	1	2	1
Base: all outpatients who used the waiting area=100%	518	486	521	308	381	1128	1086

Table 5: Proportions of patients waiting different lengths of time to be seen who found the waiting area in the department they had attended very comfortable

Patients who found the waiting area:	Time waited to be seen[1]				
	5–10 mins	about 15 mins	about 30 mins	about 45 mins	about 1 hour or more
	%	%	%	%	%
very comfortable	34	30	27	18·	15
all right	61	66	63	69	65
rather uncomfortable	4	3	8	10	16
very uncomfortable	1	1	2	3	4
Base=100%[2]	905	371	383	172	349

1. for patients who had a specific appointment time, the time waited is that beyond their actual appointment time
2. base excludes patients on stretchers or unconscious

Table 6 Proportions of patients in different age groups who were satisfied with the appearance of the waiting area in the department they had attended

The waiting area was:	Patients aged					All men	All women
	0–16	17–34	35–54	55–64	65 and over		
	%	%	%	%	%	%	%
a bright and cheerful place	34	22	36	47	51	33	40
all right	42	39	43	42	39	42	40
a bit drab and depressing	15	26	14	5	4	15	13
patient didn't take much notice	9	13	7	6	6·	10	7
Base: all outpatients who used waiting room=100%	520	486	521	306	380	1128	1085

Table 7 Proportions of patients in different social classes[1] who found the waiting area in the department they had attended very comfortable

Patients who found the waiting area:	Social class					
	I Profes- sional	II Inter- mediate	III Skilled non- manual	III Skilled manual	IV Partly skilled	V Unskilled
	%	%	%	%	%	%
very comfortable	18	21	30	27	33	43
all right	75	67	61	65	60	48
rather uncomfortable	3	10	6	7	6	8
very uncomfortable	4	2	3	1	1	1
Base: all outpatients who used the waiting area=100%	101	415	299	822	339	122

1. married women and patients aged under 16 have been classified on the basis of the head of household's occupation. All other patients have been classified on the basis of their own occupation.

Table 8 Proportions of patients in different social classes[1] who were satisfied with the appearance of the waiting area in the department they had attended

The waiting area was:	Social class					
	I Profes-sional	II Inter-mediate	III Skilled non-manual	III Skilled manual	IV Partly skilled	V Unskilled
	%	%	%	%	%	%
a bright and cheerful place	32	34	42	35	37	40
all right	41	43	36	42	40	39
a bit drab and depressing	21	16	14	14	12	9
patient didn't take much notice	6	7	8	9	11	12
Base: all outpatients who used the waiting area=100%	100	415	298	821	340	122

1. see footnote to table 7

Table 9 Proportions of outpatients who found the waiting area in the department they attended very comfortable and bright and cheerful in appearance

Patients who found the waiting area:	Patients who found the waiting area:			All
	very comfortable	all right	rather or very uncomfortable	
a bright and cheerful place	20%	15%	1%	36%
all right	6%	32%	3%	41%
drab and depressing	1%	9%	4%	14%
patient didn't take much notice	1%	8%	*	9%
All	28%	64%	8%	100%

Base: all outpatients who used the waiting area=2209=100%

Table 10 Proportions of men and women patients who were working full or part-time and who would have preferred their appointments to have been fixed for different times

Convenience of appointments	Men		Men patients of all ages	Women		Women patients of all ages
	aged 16 and over			aged 16 and over		
	working	not working		working	not working	
	%	%	%	%	%	%
appointments were usually all right	89	95	90	87	93	91
would have preferred different appointment times	11	5	10	13	7	9
Base=100%[1]	235	150	480	163	267	516

1. base=all outpatients who did not usually have a say in fixing their appointments

Table 11 The incovenience of appointments to mothers with young children

Convenience of appointments	Mother is not working and has (other) children under 11 . . .	
	patient is mother	patient is child
	%	%
appointments were usually all right	76	86
would have preferred different appointment times	24	14
Base=100%[1]	45	74

1. base=outpatients who did not usually have a say in fixing their appointments

Table 12 Reasons why patients with specific appointment times expected to have to wait to be seen at the hospital

Reasons why patients expected to have to wait	Patient expected to wait				All with specific appointment times
	about 15 mins	about 30 mins	about 45 mins	about 1 hour or longer	
	%	%	%	%	%
own previous experience	46	50	57	73	55
experience of friends/ relatives	2	3	2	4	3
common knowledge	10	12	12	5	10
time between appoint- ments too short	20	18	6	6	15
several patients given same appointment time	5	8	9	7	7
appointments made for times when doctors not available	3	4	4	6	4
many patients already waiting	22	25	22	20	23
expect serious cases to be seen first	11	8	5	6	8
hospitals short of staff	3	4	6	4	4
other answers	8	4	4	9	6
Base=100%[1] [2]	227	330	82	163	802

1. base: all outpatients with specific appointment times who expected to have to wait more than about 5 or 10 minutes after their appointment time before being seen
2. percentages add to more than 100 as some people gave more than one reason

Table 13   Reasons why patients with open appointments or no appointments at all expected to have to wait to be seen at the hospital

Reasons why patients expected to have to wait	Patients expected to wait			All
	about 15 mins	between about 30 and 40 minutes	about 1 hour or longer	
	%	%	%	%
own previous experience	29	37	58	44
experience of friends/ relatives	4	7	5	5
common knowledge	49	27	19	28
many patients already waiting	35	38	31	35
expect serious cases to be seen first	9	16	11	12
hospitals are short of staff	4	3	6	5
doctors not always available	6	4	4	4
other answers	10	3	3	5
Base=100%[1] [2]	68	135	127	330

1. base=all outpatients with open appointments or no appointments at all who expected to wait more than about 5 or 10 minutes to be seen
2. percentages add to more than 100 as some people gave more than one reason

Table 14   Outpatients' opinion of arrangements for their admission to hospital

Opinion of arrangements for admission to hospital	All outpatients[1]
	%
very satisfied	55
satisfied	35
could have been improved	10
Base=100%[1]	471

1. all outpatients who had been admitted since January 1975 to same hospital they were attending as outpatients for treatment for the same condition. Excludes those in hospital for less than 3 nights

Table 15   Outpatients' opinion of the arrangements for their discharge from hospital

Opinion of arrangements for discharge from hospital	All outpatients[1]
	%
very satisfied	50
satisfied	36
could have been improved	14
Base=100%[1]	473

1. see footnote to table 14

Table 16 Outpatients' overall opinion of the hospital inpatient service

Overall opinion of the hospital inpatient service	All outpatients[1]
	%
very good	51
good	33
has its faults	14
poor	2
Base=100%[1]	581

1. see footnote to table 14. Note this table includes those in hospital for less than 3 nights

Table 17 Proportions of outpatients who found various aspects of their treatment unpleasant and who felt they were not told enough about why they were necessary

Patients' attitudes to treatment	Treatment							
	blood sample	urine sample	injections	X-rays	physio-therapy	general anaesthetic	stitches/ clips etc	dressings done, changed, removed
	%	%	%	%	%	%	%	%
not told enough about why necessary								
and bothered	6	5	5	4	5	2	NA[1]	NA
and not bothered	26	27	13	12	7	7	NA	NA
found treatment unpleasant								
could have been made more pleasant	1	*	3	1	*	3	8	2
nothing could have been done	8	1	21	6	13	16	15	8
Base: all outpatients having treatment=100%	711	543	508	1128	245	119	275	602

1. NA=not asked

254

Table 18 Patients' overall opinion of the hospital outpatient service

Overall opinion of hospital outpatient service	Men							Women							Men and women out-patients
	0-9	10-16	17-34	35-54	55-64	65 & over	all men	0-9	10-16	17-34	35-54	55-64	65 & over	all women	
	%	%	%	%	%	%	%	%	%	%	%	%	%	%	%
very good	24	34	24	39	52	71	39	25	26	18	39	53	69	40	40
good	37	40	38	31	33	24	34	39	41	37	35	34	24	34	34
has its faults	35	25	36	26	14	5	25	33	30	41	23	13	7	24	24
poor	4	1	2	4	1	0	2	3	3	4	3	0	0	2	2
Base: all outpatients=100%	161	134	279	256	154	170	1154	135	94	224	274	159	222	1108	2262

Table 19 Proportions of patients who were told how to go about making a complaint to the Hospital Authorities should they wish to do so: those who were sent or given a hospital information booklet

Patient was . . .	All inpatients
	%
told how to go about making a complaint and . . .	
had hospital information booklet	14 } 16%
did not have information booklet	2 }
was not told how to go about making a complaint and . . .	
had hospital information booklet	45 } 84%
did not have information booklet	39 }
Base: all inpatients=100%	786

255

Table 20 Patients' overall opinion of the hospital inpatient service

Patients' overall opinion of hospital inpatient service	Men	Women maternity patients	non-maternity patients	Men and women inpatients
	%	%	%	%
very good	53	33	54	51
good	33	46	28	32
has its faults	13	20	17	16
is poor	1	1	1	1
Base: all inpatients=100%	306	97	392	795

Table 21 Proportion of inpatients who, if they had to go back into hospital again would definitely want to go into the same hospital by overall opinion of the hospital inpatient service

Whether would want to go to same hospital again	Patients' overall opinion of hospital service								All inpatients	
	very good		good		has its faults		poor			
	Nos	%	Nos	%	Nos	%	Nos	%	Nos	%
definitely would	258	33	116	15	33	4	2	*	409	52
definitely would not	11	1	10	1	26	3	5	1	52	7
wouldn't mind either way	133	17	129	16	63	8	2	*	327	41
All inpatients	402	51	255	32	122	15	9	1	Base=788	=100%

Table 22 Patients' overall opinion of the hospital inpatient service by number of nights spent in hospital

Patients' overall opinion of hospital inpatient service	Number of nights spent in hospital						All inpatients
	up to 2 nights	3–5 nights	6–7 nights	8–14 nights	15–21 nights	over 3 weeks	
	%	%	%	%	%	%	%
very good	41	44	44	57	59	64	51
good	39	33	38	30	26	28	32
has its faults	20	21	17	12	14	8	16
is poor	—	2	1	1	1	—	1
Base: all inpatients =100%	123	185	104	189	80	111	792

Table 23 Proportions of inpatients who found various aspects of their treatment unpleasant and who felt they were not told enough about why they were necessary

Patients' attitudes to treatment	Treatment							
	blood sample	urine sample	injections	X-rays	physio-therapy	general anaesthetic	stitches/ clips etc	dressings done, changed, removed
	%	%	%	%	%	%	%	%
not told enough about why necessary....								
and bothered	8	5	6	6	3	2	NA[1]	NA
and not bothered	33	31	19	17	12	16	NA	NA
found treatment unpleasant....								
could have been made more pleasant	1	1	2	1	1	*	4	1
nothing could have been done	8	1	11	5	7	6	11	7
Base: all inpatients having treatment=100%	634	554	574	389	186	410	354	287

1. NA=not asked

Printed in England for Her Majesty's Stationery Office by Robendene (Chesham) Ltd.
Dd 0586876   K 15 12/78